DIVORC

SUGAR

40 Day Sugar Detox Plan to Eliminate Sugar Cravings, Overcome Sugar Addiction, Drop Fat and Reclaim Great Health

Tina Stat

Table of Contents

Table of Contents 3

Introduction: I Am An Addict 13

    In the Beginning, There was Sugar and It was SWEET!
....17

Chapter One: Living The Sweet Life 18

    Sweet History Lesson: Where Did Sugar Come From? .19

    Food? Spice? Drug? – What Is Sugar? 20

        Sugar: ~~Anatomically~~ Molecularly Correct...................26

        Why I Became Sugar-Aware 30

Chapter Two: The Enemy Among Us 32

    The Many Aliases of Sugar – Who is on Your Label?....34

        Understanding The Label 38

    Sugar Hidden Among Your Healthy Choices 40

        Granola 40

        Protein Bars 41

        Cereal 42

        Yogurt 42

        Bread..42

        Pasta Sauce 43

        Canned or Boxed Soup 43

        Frozen Yogurt 44

        Nut and Seed Butters 45

        Sports Drinks...45

    The Difference Between Natural Sugar and Added Sugar
....46

Natural Sugars...46

Added Sugars...47

Ridding the Cabinets of Sugar.....................................47

Where Do Artificial Sweeteners Fit In?....................49

Chapter Three: What Happened To The Sweetness? 51

How Does Sugar Affect The Body? 51

Your Brain on Sugar 52

Your Mood on Sugar..52

Your Teeth on Sugar..53

Your Joints on Sugar 53

Your Skin on Sugar..53

Your Liver on Sugar...54

Your Heart on Sugar..54

Your Pancreas on Sugar 55

Your Kidneys on Sugar 55

Your Body Weight on Sugar 55

Me on Sugar...56

Five Serious Diseases That May Be Linked to Sugar 58

Cancer...58

Obesity..59

Cardiovascular Disease 59

Diabetes..60

Liver Disease..61

I Didn't Know I Was Putting My Life in Danger..........61

Proof You Are Addicted to Sweetness 63

You May Be A Sugar Addict If... 66

You Try To Hide Your Sugary Habit 66

Your Cravings Become Hard to Satisfy 67

You Eat Sugary Treats Even When You Aren't Hungry 67

You Have Constant Cravings 68

You Crave Other Foods 68

You Try To Kick The Habit, But The Withdrawal Is Too Much..69

Sugar Provides You With Emotional Support 69

Despite The Consequences, You Engage Anyway........70

You Make A Point To Get Sugar..................................70

You Feel Intense Guilt About Eating Sugar 70

My Toxic Relationship with Mr. Ose............................72

Chapter Four: The Great Sugar Exodus.............................75

The Effects of Giving Up Sugar.......................................76

Feelings of Fatigue and Weakness 77

Increased and Extreme Cravings 78

Confusion..78

Headaches...79

Changes in Behavior 79

Trouble Sleeping 80

Depression 81

Unintentional Weight Loss...81

Flu-Like Symptoms (Ketosis) 83

Periods of Lightheadedness 83

The Five Stages of Sugar Withdrawal 83

How the Withdrawal Affected Me 86

Overcoming A Sugar Addiction.......................................88

Educate Yourself 88

Be Realistic With Your Goals 89

Look For Healthy Alternatives....................................89

Turn to Protein...90

Don't Give Up...91

Exodus Invoked Changes – How Your Body Will Change
....92

Younger Looking Skin 92

Tap Into Lasting Energy...93

Reduce the Risk of Serious Health Problems 93

Doing This Now Pays Big in the Long Run................94

It Takes Time..94

Chapter Five: Detox to Break the Chains of Sugar Addiction
....96

Preparing for the Sugar Detox 97

Find a Support System 100

Restructure Your Reward System...............................101

Accept That You Might Fail 101

Prepare to Put in the Time and Effort.......................102

Do Not Approach This as Easy 102

Exercise Through the Withdrawal...............................103

How Does Exercise Help?...103

Get Your Confidence Back...104

Get More Social..105

Healthy Coping Mechanism 105

"Exercise" Isn't Always Exercise 106

How To Get Started Boosting Yourself Through Exercise 107

Honesty is the Best Policy - *Author Confession* 109

Using Meditation 109

Using Yoga...114

Building Your Yoga Sequence 117

Strength Training 119

Aerobic Exercises 121

Just Be Active...125

Chapter Six: A 40-Day Sugar Detox Plan 126

The Birth of a Plan 128

Making Changes To Reduce Sugar 132

Stop Drinking Your Sugar 132

What Increasing Protein Can Do During Sugar Detox 133

Include Healthy High-Fat Foods 135

Choose Fresh Fruit and Vegetables in a Pinch..........136

Reach for Healthy Snacks 137

Stage 1: Days 1-10..138

Setting Goals 139

Choosing Positive Self-Affirmations 140

Start a Journal 142

Better Days Will Come.......................................142

Stage 2: Days 11-20 144

Make Your Goals a Tad Harder 144

Maintain Healthy Eating Habits 145

Keep Up with Your Journal, Blog, Vlog, Whatever!...145

Increase Your Physical Activity 146

Stage 3: Days 21-30 147

    Decide on a Big Goal for Day 40 147

    Create Your Stage 3 Goals 148

    Talk About Your Experiences 149

Stage 4: Days 31-40 150

    Don't Quit Because You Feel Ahead 150

    Start Thinking About the Future 151

    Constantly Acknowledge the Home Stretch 152

Stage 5: Days 41+Beyond 154

    How to Create a Plan Going Forward 155

    My 40-Day Detox 156

Do It For Yourself 157

Chapter Seven: Recipes, Snacks, and Making It 162

Breakfast Recipes 165

    Cottage Cheese Pancakes 166

    PB Cup Smoothie 167

    Paleo Minute English Muffins 168

    No Egg Breakfast Bake 169

    Cheesy Egg Muffins with Green Chiles 171

    Shamrock Breakfast Sandwich 172

    Simple Breakfast Hash 174

    Egg White Frittata 176

    Black Forest Turkey with Egg Cups 178

    Clean Eating Black Bean Scramble 179

Lunch Recipes 180

    Greek Orzo Salad 181

Grilled Buffalo Chicken in Lettuce Wraps 183

BLT Chicken Salad...185

Garden Frittata 187

Cauliflower Pizza Lunch Muffins 189

Turkey Pesto Cucumber Roll-ups 191

Cold Lemon Zoodles 192

Nori Vegetable Rolls 193

Spinach Stuffed Cremini Mushrooms with Feta........194

Avocado Egg Salad..196

Dinner Recipes 197

Rosemary Garlic Pork Tenderloin............................198

Lamb Kofta Kebab 200

Mexican Skillet Zucchini...202

Grilled Garlic and Herb Chicken with Vegetables.....204

Lime and Garlic Marinated Pork Chops...................206

Zoodles with Pesto and Tomatoes 208

Skillet Steak with Mushrooms and Onions 209

Rosemary Broiled Salmon 211

Chicken and Avocado Soup 213

Roasted Broccoli Parmesan 215

Pass on Dessert...217

Keeping Your Meal Planning Simple 217

Try New Things..218

Fridge, Freezer, and Pantry Staples...............................218

Refrigerator...219

Freezer 220

Pantry Essentials 221

Buy a Little Here – Buy a Little There 225

Learning How to Make It 226

Anxiety Driven Marketing.............................226

Cravings and Addiction Through Advertising 227

Even Television Lures You In...........................227

Recognize and Move Forward 228

Change Your Surroundings 229

Bittersweet Facts About Sugar 229

Chapter Eight: The Truth, The Whole Truth, and Nothing But The Truth (About...) 233

The Truth About Obesity.................................233

Three Classes of Obesity 234

Causes of Obesity.......................................235

Is There a Cure?...235

The Truth About Type 2 Diabetes 235

Symptoms Associated with Type 2 Diabetes 236

Risk Factors of Developing Type 2 Diabetes 236

Consequences of Type 2 Diabetes....................238

The Truth About High Blood Pressure....................239

High Blood Pressure Can Lead to These Serious Diseases 239

Understanding Your Blood Pressure.................240

What Do These Have in Common?....................241

The Villian in the Scenario.............................242

Be an Overcomer 243

Roll with the Punches – There will be a lot! 243

Conclusion: There is Life After Sugar....................245

Your Body, Your Choice 245

   Think About Your Current Health 246

   Do This For Yourself 247

Why You Need to Sugar Detox 247

   Don't Give Up 248

Download The Audiobook Free!

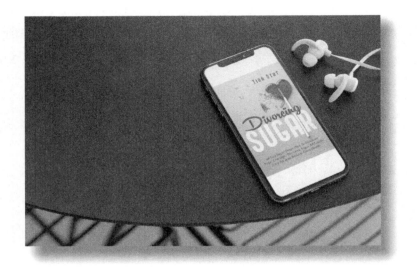

Just to say thanks I would like to give you the
audiobook version 100% free!

To get instant free access go to:
http://www.tinastat.com/audiobook

Introduction: I Am An Addict

Sugar is the sociopath of foods. It acts sweet...but it's really poison. -Karen Salmansohn

I am an addict, but not in the way you may think. My addiction is sugar. Correction, my addiction *was* sugar. The funny thing about addiction is that once you have one, you always struggle with it. I'm not alone, though. Others are out there – many just haven't come to terms with it.

I don't know when I realized that sugar had a hold on my life. I just know that I was craving it constantly and would make impromptu trips to the store to satisfy it. The more you crave it, the more you eat to satisfy the craving. At some point, you spiral out of control.

Simply put, sugar is a class of sweet-tasting carbohydrates. Despite being a fuel for the brain, sugar is also viewed as a reward, making you want more. The more you put your brain in reward mode, the more it will want it, and the habit will be harder to break. Let's look at what being addicted means and how it can relate to sugar:

Addicts *may* have impulsive behavior – being impulsive sporadically is common, but those who cannot control these actions are more likely to form addictions as a result. *Have you ever sat and eaten the entire pint of ice cream without intending to because you couldn't stop?*

Addicts *may* be compulsive – compulsion is when habits and behaviors are repeated on a cycle that cannot be broken without an intervention. *"This is the last candy bar I'm eating, "only to repeat the habit the next day with the same promises.*

Addicts *may* have problems handling stress – it is funny to think that not eating a candy bar could make it impossible to handle stress. Many people turn to food or other sweets to handle stress. *Stress eating, anyone?*

Addicts *may* suffer from low self-esteem – some addicts turn to their "drug" to create better feelings about themselves. For example, the increase in dopamine during a sugar rush or high can create improved feelings.

Addicts *may* be in denial – addicts who do not know they have a problem may be in denial about the entire situation. *"I don't have a problem, and I can stop whenever I want. "*

How can sugar be so sweet but as harmful as an illicit drug just like cocaine?

Sweet Medicine or Illicit Drug?

It seems like a long-shot to compare sugar to cocaine, right? I'm not the first one to make this comparison. Both were initially used for medicinal purposes throughout history – prohibition ended the cocaine reign (more or less).

When sugar was first introduced in ancient Greece and Rome, it was used as medicine and in the wealthiest patrons" food. Sugar dates back to 8000 BCE when indigenous people of New Guinea chewed it raw.

Cocaine also has a medicinal history but is now illegal in the United States. Just like sugar, cocaine is derived from a plant, the coca plant, to be exact. For centuries, the coca plant (derived as cocaine) was used for medicines. Even your favorite Coke used it as an ingredient at one time. Prohibition put a stop to a lot of the substances that caused altered states, not just alcohol.

How can one addictive substance be legal and another one not?

Both of these chemicals have effects on the brain, changing the way the body feels. Sugar can give you a temporary energy rush – a stimulant effect. Drugs are often referred to as uppers or downers. Cocaine is an upper – a stimulant.

Coincidence that both of these are highly addictive substances?

So, what can you do to break an addiction to cocaine? Rehabilitation? The first step to a drug rehabilitation program is detox, followed by support. Yes, sugar rehabilitation does exist, but utilizing the right steps of sugar detox on your own can be just as beneficial and satisfying.

Sugar Detox

By definition, detox is the removal of toxic substances from the living body. Detox comes with a price, mostly if not done correctly. Side effects of withdrawal can be intense – so intense that these symptoms discourage addicts from giving up the substance. I'm not just talking about hard street drugs. I'm talking about sugar, too. Sugar can make your body go crazy when suddenly denied it when you are an addict. Detox is not impossible, which you are going to find out as you read along. You are going to find out exactly what I learned – sugar is a hidden enemy.

In the Beginning, There was Sugar and It was SWEET!

How often do you think about when you first came into contact with sugar? What is your earliest memory of tasting those granules on your tongue? Maybe it wasn't even pure sugar, it could have been a cookie from a neighbor or even a cupcake treat during a birthday party. Either way, you probably don't remember when it happened.

I don't remember when it happened, I just remember sugar always being readily available. Not just any sugar, refined sugar. When you do a good job in school, you get candy. Halloween, Valentines, Christmas – CANDY! Some dentists will even give you a "sugar-free" lollipop after a good cleaning. Why has the world gone mad?

You Can Fight The Feeling

For the sake of your health, we are going to work through your addiction to sugar together. Through planning your meals and making your grocery lists to stocking your cabinets with the right stuff. You are the only one who will sabotage your efforts. Let this book and my story be your guide through this new world.

Chapter One: Living The Sweet Life

Sugar may have had an impact on your body before you were born. As a fetus in your mother's womb – you were exposed to sugar. Mothers who experience high blood sugar levels during pregnancy, also known as gestational diabetes, can cause problems after birth. Since the fetus was used to the high levels of sugar from the blood, the baby can be born with hypoglycemia because of the lack of sugar after.

If this wasn't a problem for your mother before birth, it was inevitable that you were exposed to sugar after you were born. "Breast is best" is the common reference made after you have a baby. Breast milk contains all the nutrients your baby needs. There is no denying that. It also contains sugar, though.

If you weren't breastfed as a baby, that means you had formula. Guess what? Your body was exposed to sugar here too. Not all sugar is bad when consumed in limited quantities, so don't think that you are exposing your child to something dangerous.

The point that I am trying to make to you is that we are all exposed to sugar from a very young age. We will inevitably acquire a taste for sugar at some point in our lives. How we handle it will determine how it affects our lives.

Sweet History Lesson: Where Did Sugar Come From?

Sugar can be traced back as far as 8000 BCE (before the current era) when the indigenous people of New Guinea chewed it raw. From 8000 BCE through 600 CE (current era), sugar cane cultivation practices spread through Southeast Asia, China, and India through various trade routes.

In 350 AD, the Indians are the ones who are responsible for discovering how to crystallize the substance. After sharing this secret with traveling Buddhist Monks, the methods were shared with China. Three hundred years later, it became a staple in the culinary arts of India, the Middle East, and China.

Sugar cane plantations soon popped up across the world, which was facilitated by the transatlantic slave trade. The use of slaves for the mass crop cultivations finally ended in 1888 in Great Britain and the United States. During this time, the discovery was made by Andrea S. Margraff discovered that the root of the beet could be used for sugar extraction. The sugar beet came to America in 1838 but was not used commercially for sugar until 1870.

The 20th century saw a massive increase in sugar production, and in 1907 the Domino Sugar brand was born. Domino Sugar was the company responsible for the majority of the United States' sugar production and distribution.

Food? Spice? Drug? — What Is Sugar?

How about all three? Sugar is used in foods and is also used to enhance like a spice. It was once used medicinally and is still added to some medications. How are you supposed to handle this triple threat?

Something to understand is that all green plants use photosynthesis to create sugar. Photosynthesis is a process used by green plants and some other organisms. It allows for the plant or organism to convert light energy into chemical energy.

Step One: The plant or organism pulls water and minerals from the ground. In the case of green plants, it uses its roots.

Step Two: Leaves absorb carbon dioxide that is in the air.

Step Three: Energy from the sun is absorbed by chlorophyll in the leaves.

Step Four: The energy from the sunlight makes sucrose from carbon dioxide and water.

As you might have guessed, sugar cane and sugar beets have the highest sugar quantity out of all plants. The sugars you find within these are the same type of pure sweetness you find in fruits and vegetables.

Although not considered a spice anymore, sugar was historically referred to as one. Sugar is appealing like a spice. It creates a sweet flavor and is commonly presented in a way that seems non-threatening.

Look at this version of *"What Are Little Girls Made Of?"*
The referenced version is from *The Baby's Opera* by Walter
Crane and circa 1877.

Verse 1:

"What are little boys made of?
What are little boys made of?
Frogs and snails and puppy-dog's tails,
And that are little boys made of."

Verse 2:

"What are little girls made of?
What are little girls made of?
Sugar and spice and all that's nice,
And that are little girls made of."

Verse 3:

"What are young men made of?
What are young men made of?
Sighs and leers, and crocodile tears,
And that are young men made of."

Verse 4:

"What are young women made of?
What are young women made of?
Ribbons and laces, and sweet pretty faces,
And that are young women made of."

From early in history, sugar was referenced not only as
edible but as a description. Sugar was depicted as
something pleasant. During this time, little girls and young
women did not have rights and were not empowered like

they are today. Back then, they were considered delicate and pleasant – compliant. They were sweet, sweet as sugar.

So how does sugar fit into different industries? Sugar has versatile uses, which span across the health industry, beauty industry, home and garden, and the industrial and agricultural markets.

Health Industry

- Used to create a coating, add volume or texture, and can flavor medications. Sugar can also be used as a preservative or an antioxidant.
- Sugar can stop the hiccups by the phrenic nerves to reset due to the grainy texture that slightly irritates the esophagus.
- You can relieve painful bug bites or stings using equal parts of water and sugar and applying the mixture to the area. Leave it for about 20 minutes.
- Spicy or hot food sensations in the mouth can be relieved by sucking on a pinch of sugar or a sugar cube.
- Ease a sore throat by using a candy or lozenge to increase saliva, keeping your throat moistened and alleviating the irritation.
- Some studies show babies given a 1 to 4 sugar and water solution handled the pain from their immunizations better than those who only had water.
- The use of sugar on open wounds has been found to help with the healing process by removing the excess moisture to make the area bacteria resistant.

Beauty Industry

- Sugar is often added to cosmetic products for exfoliating and moisturizing.
- If you sprinkle sugar on your lips after applying lipstick, it will make the color last longer.
- Body scrubs and lip scrubs containing sugar are becoming popular because of the moisturizing and exfoliating properties.

Home and Garden

- Using sugar to clean your hands can help remove grease and acts as an abrasive to remove other substances.
- A pretreating agent made of water, white vinegar, and sugar can be placed on stains for up to 20 minutes to help with the removal process.
- Add sugar cubes to an airtight container that is holding baked goods. It will remove the moisture and keep the items fresher for longer.
- Flowers stay fresher longer when put in a vase with three teaspoons of sugar and two tablespoons of vinegar per one quart of water. The sugar feeds your flower stems while the vinegar keeps bacteria from growing. Replace every other day for a longer-lasting flower arrangement.
- Sugar can be used to make effective indoor and outdoor pest solutions.

Industrial and Agricultural

- Sugar cane bagasse is used in the production of particleboard.
- Sugar cane is used in the production of bioplastics that are used in a variety of capacities.
- Sugar cane bagasse is used to make office products and take-out containers, which are eco-friendlier than Styrofoam.
- The coproducts of sugar production and molasses are used as supplemental feeding for livestock.
- Sugar is used to slow down the setting time of cement and glue.
- Sugar is used in the production of biofuels.

Sugar: ~~Anatomically~~ Molecularly Correct

The scientific name used to describe sugar is sucrose. Sucrose is a molecule created by the grouping of 12 carbon atoms, 22 hydrogen atoms, and 11 oxygen atoms. For all intents and purposes, anything created from a combination of these three atoms is considered to be a carbohydrate.

$$C_{12}H_{22}O_{11}$$

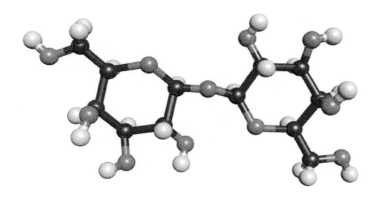

Sucrose is made from two smaller molecules, glucose and fructose. An acidic, like lemon juice, can break up this molecule into glucose and fructose. There are two types of carbohydrates, simple sugars and starches. Simple sugars include fructose, glucose, and lactose, to name a few. Within this carbohydrate group is naturally occurring sugars and added sugars.

The human body doesn't understand the difference between the sugar in an apple and the sugar in a cupcake. Both types are metabolized in the body the same way. Your ability to tell the difference between natural sugar and an added sugar can make all the difference. Added sugar equals extra calories.

It may come as a shock to you that a lot of us sugar addicts are obese. Type 2 diabetes is also a risk factor for us as well, but that's another chapter. This chapter is about understanding sugar – scientifically.

Sugars can be:

Monosaccharides – a single molecular structure that is absorbed directly into the bloodstream, such as glucose, fructose, galactose, and mannose

Disaccharides – two molecules are placed together to create sugars broken down into the body into two different sugars

Example:

Sugar	Molecule 1	Molecule 2
Sucrose	Glucose	Fructose
Lactose	Glucose	Galactose
Maltose	Glucose	Glucose
Trehalose*	Glucose	Glucose

*different molecular composition of the two glucose molecules

Polysaccharides – ten or more monosaccharide molecules, which creates starch

With the new research that has been done regarding added sugar, food manufacturers were required to change the food product labels to include the amount of added sugar in the item. The ***Dietary Guidelines for Americans 2015-2020*** recommend that people consume less than 10% of their calorie consumption from added sugars.

Let's put this into a little better perspective:

1g of sugar = 4 calories

4g of sugar = 1 teaspoon

Suppose you decide that you have watched what you ate all day long so that you can have a snack cake before bed. You know the snack cakes I'm talking about, comes in a box, crème filling, the ones that literally melt in your mouth.

Before you get side swept away with the idea of this snack cake, I want to pick it apart. On average, these have about 200 calories and include 19g of sugar. Given what we know about calories and grams of sugar – suppose you follow a strict 1200 calorie diet for weight loss purposes. That means, per guidelines, you should only have 30g per day of added sugar. The Heart Association recommends 25g per 1200 calories.

I hate to send your world crashing down around you, but that snack cake is taking up 19g of that 30g total. Is it worth it?

Why I Became Sugar-Aware

Added sugar is one of the largest culprits of weight gain and obesity. If you are like me, you drank most of your calories. Regular soda, juice, and sweetened teas are full of sugar. Depending on the soda you find yourself most acquainted with, you could be ranging from 30 to 50 grams of sugar per serving.

I've spent most of my life addicted to sugar. A lot of it was without realizing I was, too. I never understood why I kept gaining weight and why no amount of exercise was working. There was that "ah-ha" moment when I woke up one morning, and I needed my caffeine, which came in the form of a soda.

Why was I relying so heavily on this? Because I was addicted to the sugar and the extra kick, it provided the caffeine. I drank more of it during the day when my energy levels started to decrease – I wanted that jolt to wake me up.

I started looking into patterns, not just of my drinks but also my food, and I found something rather alarming. The rate at which I was feeding my body sugar was unbelievable. Furthermore, I was doing it without any regard for myself, my health, or my self-esteem.

I began keeping track to see where I could cut down on the sugar, but it was lurking behind every dark corner. What was I supposed to do?

That was when I knew I had to develop an attack plan.

Chapter Two: The Enemy Among Us

Sugar is the secret double agent of the carbohydrate brigade. Besides being beautifully crafted and enticing, it also hides in plain sight, using names that none of us common folk understand. You can look at a three-tier cake covered in edible glitter confetti and gleaming under the lights and know the size of the sugar high that would follow.

The secret agent in your fridge is the ketchup. Most tomato-based condiments and sauces are full of sugar due to the product's acidity. The use of sucrose weakens this acidity. There are almost 4g of sugar in one tablespoon of ketchup (you know you aren't *only* eating one tablespoon either).

The rule is moderation – how much sugar is enough, and how much is too much? I don't know about you, but moderation was never one of my particular skills. I spent a lot of time fueling sugar into this body, and the idea of cutting down slightly appalled me. How would I cut this out of my diet when I've already brought it to this point?

What I didn't realize at the time was that no one was telling me that I had to give up sugar completely. I just needed to bring it to a healthy level. So how was I going to eliminate the excess sugar in my diet?

I started doing my research on the subject. Knowledge is power, after all. That was when I found out about the various aliases that sugar uses. These are often found buried deep in your nutritional label.

The Many Aliases of Sugar – Who is on Your Label?

Sugar wears many different cloaks and has a pocket full of aliases it uses. Some of its names are obvious, but others don't stand out as noticeably. It is estimated that 76% of added sugar is hidden in the packaged foods you purchase at the store.

Monosaccharides and disaccharides are the most commonly used names you might find on a label. These are simple sugars and are composed of their own unique molecular compounds containing carbon, hydrogen, and oxygen atoms.

- Dextrose
- Fructose
- Galactose
- Glucose
- Lactose
- Maltose
- Sucrose

The next set of sugars are often found solid or in granulated forms. These may be added into products or simply sold on their own.

- Beet Sugar
- Brown Sugar
- Cane Sugar
- Cane Juice Crystals
- Coconut Sugar

- Castor Sugar
- Corn Syrup Solids
- Confectioner's Sugar (powdered sugar)
- Date Sugar
- Crystalline Fructose
- Demerara Sugar
- Diastatic Malt
- Dextrin
- Ethyl Maltol
- Golden Sugar
- Florida Crystals
- Grape Sugar
- Glucose Sugar Solids
- Maltodextrin
- Icing Sugar
- Panela Sugar
- Muscovado Sugar
- Granulated Table Sugar
- Yellow Sugar
- Sucanat
- Turbinado Sugar

Sugars can also come in liquid or syrup forms. You will find these more in cooking or food-related items.

- Agave Nectar/Syrup
- Blackstrap Molasses
- Barley Malt
- Buttered Sugar (buttercream)
- Brown Rice Syrup
- Carob Syrup
- Caramel
- Corn Syrup

- Fruit Juice
- Evaporated Can Juice
- Fruit Juice Concentrate
- High-Fructose Corn Syrup
- Golden Syrup
- Honey
- Malt Syrup
- Invert Sugar
- Rice Syrup
- Molasses
- Maple Syrup
- Sorghum Syrup
- Refiner's Syrup
- Treacle

These sugars can often be found in foods, drinks, and prepackaged items. You may see the name of some of these sugars and know precisely what foods or beverages they are in. Others might be a little harder to guess.

I was amazed at the number of products that had sugars hidden within them when I started doing my research. Items that I had used my entire life were a significant source of added sugar. Added sugars are not conducive to daily living. They have no nutritional value.

Cookies, Cakes, Pastries – Surely, this was a given for added sugar. The sheer composition of these is based on a foundation of sugar, with sugar, and topped with sugar. These are often weaknesses because they are appealing to the eye, but they taste just as exquisite.

36

Bread, Pasta, Crackers – I wouldn't have thought about bread, pasta, or crackers having added sugar. Sure, these are high in carbohydrates – which are also sugar. I never put two and two together, mostly since pasta was a staple part of my diet.

Beverages – Beverages from milk to soda can have added sugar in them. The term "drinking your calories" comes from the fact that you are drinking nothing but added sugar. You can create a lot of health problems by drinking all your calories on top of eating them.

Salad Dressing, Condiments – Some salad dressings and condiments have a lot of sugar in them. I already talked about ketchup, but BBQ sauce is another that has high levels of sugar added.

Yogurt – Why!? The betrayal! Trying to get healthy, yogurt seems like a logical choice – but it is full of added sugar. All yogurt isn't bad. You just have to know how to be label-conscious.

Understanding The Label

Light. Natural. Multigrain. Low-Calorie. No Added Sugar.
Labels can read several things, but it doesn't always mean
that they are correct. The most common claims for
packaged food are:

- **Light:** Light products are manufactured or
  processed to reduce either calories or fat. Some of
  the products are watered down (think ranch dressing
  – definitely a difference in the consistency). See if
  sugar has been added to help reduce the fat or
  calories.
- **Multigrain:** Despite sounding healthy, the
  deception comes from the presence of more than one
  grain. These grains are more than likely refined.
  Whole grain is healthier than multigrain.
- **Natural** – Natural can be used on labels if natural
  products were used at some point in the process.
- **Organic** – Organic does not always mean that
  something is healthy. Organic is a process. Organic
  sugar is still metabolized like regular cane sugar.
- **No Added Sugar** – Just because there is no added
  sugar content doesn't mean that the product wasn't
  naturally high in sugar, to begin with. It also means
  that unhealthy sugar substitutes could have been
  used to compensate.

The serving size is often an area that is ignored. Serving
sizes come in all shapes, sizes, and quantities. You may
think that you happened upon a great sugar save,
something like 2g of sugar. Later you realized that mistakes
were made. Basically, after eating the whole box, you see

serving size – three pieces and servings per box – 10. Needless to say, 60g of added sugar later, you aren't feeling too hot about yourself.

Been there. Done that. Writing the book about it!

The serving size isn't the only thing you need to understand on a nutritional label. The ingredients list lets you feel like Sherlock Holmes, following the clues to determine if you are, in fact staring at the unhealthy culprit.

A little tidbit of advice – **A product's ingredients are listed by the ingredients' quantity, from highest to lowest.**

If you look at the first three ingredients and they are comprised of **refined grains**, some type of **sugar**, or **hydrogenated oil**, it can be safely assumed that the product is not the healthiest option for you.

The healthiest choice is to use products where **whole foods** are used in the first three ingredients.

Sugar and its many aliases should be an afterthought on your ingredient label, not on the forefront.

Sugar Hidden Among Your Healthy Choices

You have decided to start eating healthier. When I decided that enough was enough, and I was going to start being more food conscious, I did the same thing. I started looking up foods considered "healthy" – you can't go wrong with that Google search, right? I began by creating a menu and eating plan for the weeks ahead.

Little did I know that I was creating a menu high in added sugar, consuming just as much, if not more than I was before. Maybe it is all just a conspiracy set in motion by those covert sugar agents that creep around, rearing their ugly heads into the foods of people everywhere. How can you identify where sugar hides in your healthy choices?

Granola

We often look at granola, and our mind shouts, "health food!" Which at first glance, that would be your mind's assumption, but heavy-handed add-ins often create large amounts of sugar in impossible serving sizes. I call these serving sizes impossible because they usually run from an eighth of a cup to a quarter of a cup – can you suffice with only that much granola?

When looking at the label, my suggestion is to look at the serving size and adjust your totals based on how much you would eat. Realistically, you are more likely to eat half to one full cup, so the amount of added sugar you might be consuming will possibly be in the double digits.

Possible secret sugar agents to watch for:

- Brown rice syrup
- Molasses
- Corn syrup
- Rice malt syrup
- Evaporated cane juice

Protein Bars

First and foremost, the thing to remember is that not all protein bars are created equal. Most protein bars are used for after workout refueling. Still, others are nothing more than a candy bar with some added protein content. Beware the imposters as they may seem healthy and wholesome but are full of sugars like:

- Cane syrup
- Brown rice syrup
- Cane invert syrup

These are often added to enhance flavor, but being aware of sugar alcohols such as glycerin, which are used to keep the sugar content low but have no nutritional value themselves. Always look to the protein bars with over 20 grams of protein, but check the sugar content.

Cereal

Cereal is a universal breakfast food. There are so many different kinds of cereal, from gluten-free to sugar-free, and even different types of grains or fruits. Sadly, most cereals are full of added sugar.

We have all fallen prey to the easiness of cereal. Not sure what to have for supper? Eat a bowl of cereal. Are you looking for a quick snack? Eat a bowl of cereal. You have to be on high alert for sugar with cereal, including:

- Plain sugar
- Brown sugar syrup
- Fruit juice
- Dextrose
- And many other types of sugar additives

Yogurt

Most yogurt can be considered a healthy choice, even with a decent amount of sugar when the fruit is included. Fructose is a naturally occurring sugar that is found in fruit. The sugar that is found in yogurt and is listed before any fruit would be considered added sugar. Many times, sugar is added to low-fat yogurt to help enhance the taste that is lost when fats are removed.

Bread

You may assume that specialty loaves of bread like honey nut or cranberry might be full of added sugar, but you may not realize that white and wheat varieties can also have these additional sugars added.

Potential sugars found on labels, hiding in plain sight, are molasses, evaporated cane juice, high fructose corn syrup, and fruit juice concentrates.

When you look at the bare necessities of bread, you left with flour, water, salt, and yeast. The ones made with whole grains are considered the best. You should be wary of bread that has more than 2 grams of sugar per slice. They likely have a lot of added sugar content.

Pasta Sauce

It is not unusual for pasta sauce recipes to have some sugar to bring out the tomatoes' sweetness and cut down the acidity. The problem for added sugar comes in the sauces that are jarred. You won't likely find a label that boasts zero grams of sugar. The reason is that tomatoes have sugar in them naturally. When sugar is added to tomato-based sauces, it is usually listed as sugar on the ingredients and easily spotted. Try to steer clear of any sauce that has over seven grams of sugar.

Canned or Boxed Soup

You might be surprised by the amount of sugar hiding in your favorite soups. Soup is often great for those nights when you are running low on time or when the weather is cold. Sadly, these can come with a lot of added sugars. Look at the ingredients for:

- Cane sugar
- Sugar
- Evaporated cane juice
- High fructose corn syrup

Some soups are likely to have a higher sugar content than others, such as tomato, butternut squash, sweet potato, minestrone, and carrot, among other varieties.

Frozen Yogurt

Frozen yogurt is marketed as a healthier alternative to ice cream, citing less fat and a more delectable texture. Unfortunately, where frozen yogurt lacks in fat, it makes up in sugar. When you are in a self-serve setting, you are likely to eat more than one serving, which means multiple grams of added sugar.

You will find sugar in the form of:

- Cane sugar
- Corn syrup
- Fructose
- Sucralose
- Malitol syrup
- Fruit concentrates

Even before you add all the fun toppings and flavors, you are looking at a base of 17 to 25 grams of sugar per half cup of frozen yogurt.

Nut and Seed Butters

Butters made from peanuts, sunflower kernels, cashews, and almonds are healthy because they give good fats and proteins. There are a lot of brands that put a lot of added sugar in their products. Some of those claiming to be all-natural will try to enhance the flavor by incorporating hidden sugars. Even reduced fat ones add sugar. Look for cane syrup, dextrose, and palm sugar.

Sports Drinks

The purpose of sports drinks is to replenish the fluids and electrolytes lost during strenuous activity. For this reason, a little bit of sugar is good, but most of these include way more added sugar than necessary. The sugars present in these drinks will be listed as dextrose, sucrose, maltodextrin, and fructose. Some of the brands even opt for high fructose corn syrup. If you need to replenish electrolytes, using coconut water is an excellent alternative.

The Difference Between Natural Sugar and Added Sugar

Natural sugars and added sugars are different. I didn't know that in the beginning. I only was under the assumption that there wasn't a different – sugar is sugar, right? But there is a big difference between the two, and understanding that distinction can mean the difference between consuming too much added sugar.

Natural Sugars

The natural sugars are the ones that occur naturally in the foods you eat and the drinks you drink. The whole foods that contain these natural sugars provide additional benefits that include fiber and antioxidants.

An example of natural sugar is fructose. In the natural form, fructose is what gives fruits their sugary and natural taste. Our bodies take the fructose we eat and store the calories as fat for use as energy later. When we eat fructose, it comes with additional fiber and water content that helps us feel full.

Some processed foods add fructose that has been removed from their natural sources. We don't feel full in this form, which causes us to eat repeatedly and in larger quantities. The fructose that we overload on in this form can cause more fat to be stored, causing obesity problems.

Added Sugars

Added sugars are grouped into a category as any sugar that is not naturally occurring in a substance, typically food. Added sugars often turn into fat and cause obesity in those consuming it. The risk factors for health conditions increase with the presence of a disease or condition, especially if that person is overweight.

When you are looking at the additional sugars added to a food or beverage, the important thing is that they have NO NUTRITIONAL VALUE.

Ridding the Cabinets of Sugar

I remember finding all this information out about sugar. How was I going to make the necessary changes? I looked at my refrigerator and my pantry – it was appalling. Even when I was making an effort to eat right I was shooting myself in the foot. Trust me, it's hard to exercise without both feet.

What exactly was I going to do with all this food? I didn't want to just throw it in the garbage, that seemed like a waste.

Then it hit me. Changing my lifestyle to sugar-free was my choice and not everyone shares that same view on the issue. So, I boxed it all up, including anything unopened from my fridge and I took it to the local food pantry. Someone was bound to appreciate it and by throwing it away I could be wasting food that someone potentially needed. If you decide to purge your pantry, fridge, and cabinets, I recommend talking to your church or local food bank about donating.

Where Do Artificial Sweeteners Fit In?

Artificial sweeteners are also known as sugar substitutes. These are chemicals added to foods and beverages to make them sweeter. Some find that these taste up to several thousands of times sweeter than sugar.

Despite the calories that may be included in these sweeteners, the amount needed is so small that they are often marketed as "zero-calorie" sweeteners. The sweeteners don't calculate any of the calories because of the minuscule amount required to create the sweet taste.

Common artificial sweeteners you will see on labels are:

- Aspartame – sold under the brand names NutraSweet, Sugar Twin, and Equal, is up to 200 times sweeter than regular table sugar.
- Acesulfame potassium – also known as acesulfame K, is 200 times sweeter than sugar and is often used to cook and bake. Brand names include Sweet One and Sunnet.
- Advantame – this artificial sweetener is 20,000 times sweeter than sugar and is best suited for baking and cooking.
- Cyclamate – this artificial sweetener is 50 times sweeter than regular sugar but has been banned in the United States since 1970.
- Saccharin – the most commonly used name is Sweet'N Low, Sweet Twin, or Necta Sweet. It is 700 times sweeter than table sugar.

- Sucralose – sold under the common brand name Splenda, sucralose is 600 times sweeter than regular sugar.

There are conflicting studies on the effects of artificial sweeteners on the human body. Many people choose to use it when trying to lose weight because they are a zero-calorie alternative. Some people who have diabetes prefer to use artificial sweeteners because they do not metabolize it like regular sugar.

Some of the symptoms that artificial sweeteners cause in people are what make them detest them. The link between headaches, depression, and seizures has been discovered in some people who used these sweeteners.

There have been links to aspartame affecting people who have mood disorders, increasing the depression symptoms.

Chapter Three: What Happened To The Sweetness?

Did you know that sugar can cause harm to the body? Too much of a good thing can cause short-term or long-term health problems. Hearing that blew my mind. Why in the world would something that is naturally occurring reak so much havoc on the body? I wanted to find out what sugar can do to the body and why we are so aloof to the dangers. You don't hear a lot about these problems, at least being directly linked – that's where my mission found its purpose.

How Does Sugar Affect The Body?

You probably already know by this point that sugar is bad, at least in mass quantities. If it wasn't, then why would we be going through this exploration of sugar detox together? I wanted to find out what all these sugary candies, baked goods, drinks, and all the other alluring sugary delectables on the market today were about.

No matter how you look at the label, sugar is sugar. Your body identifies it in the same way, natural or added. The more added sugar you put in your diet, the more likely you are to experience the adverse effects.

Your Brain on Sugar

When you eat sugar, your brain gets a surge of dopamine. Dopamine is a "feel-good" chemical within your brain. Added sugars tend to release more dopamine than natural sugars. That is why your body is more likely to crave a sugary treat in the middle of the day for a pick me up versus a piece of fruit.

Once your brain starts releasing the dopamine from the added sugars, it will crave it and need more to be satisfied. You are likely to see that you begin craving sugar when your body begins to hit a "low." Then you fall into the trap of satisfying it by giving in, which soon becomes a habit that is hard to kick.

Your Mood on Sugar

Sugar causes your body's blood sugar levels to rise rapidly, giving you the intense burst of energy you crave. As your blood cells absorb the sugar, you are on course for the sugar crash, which is often signaled by jitteriness and anxiety. To stave these feelings, you may begin eating sugar to keep those reactions from happening. Studies have shown that high sugar intake can be a cause of depression in adults.

Your Teeth on Sugar

Your dentist's words ringing through your ears, warning you that candy will rot your teeth, weren't a folk story. Bacteria is what causes cavities and decay in your teeth. Guess what the favorite meal of this bacteria is – that's right, sugar. The more sugar you eat, the more susceptible you are to cavities unless you brush after every serving.

Your Joints on Sugar

Most joint pain can be attributed to inflammation. Excess amounts of sugar consumption can cause inflammation. Plus, there are even studies that show eating large amounts of sugar could increase the likelihood of developing rheumatoid arthritis.

Your Skin on Sugar

Sugary inflammation does more than just harm your joints. It can also cause you to age prematurely. When excess sugar attaches to the proteins in your bloodstream, it can create harmful moles called advanced glycation end products (AGEs). These moles have been shown to damage your collagen and the elastin in your skin, creating wrinkles and saggy skin.

Your Liver on Sugar

Your liver is in charge of processing fructose. While it is naturally occurring, it is also one of the sugars extracted and used as an added sugar. When too much fructose or high fructose corn syrup passes through the liver, it can actually damage it. When the liver breaks down the fructose, it is turned into fat.

- No-alcoholic fatty liver disease (NAFLD) is caused when there is excess fat built-up in the liver.
- Non-alcoholic steatohepatitis (NASH) is when scarring occurs on the liver. This scarring can cause the blood supply to be cut off from the liver, causing cirrhosis and a possible need for a transplant.

Your Heart on Sugar

The more sugar you eat, the more insulin gets released into your bloodstream. Insulin can affect your arteries by causing inflammation that makes them grow thicker and stiffer. Over time the stress can damage the heart or lead to heart disease. Research suggests that eating less sugar can lower blood pressure, lowering the risk factors for heart disease and heart failure.

Your Pancreas on Sugar

When insulin is released into your bloodstream, it comes from the pancreas. The more sugar you eat, the harder your pancreas has to work. If you overwork your pancreas by eating massive amounts of sugar regularly, you could be at risk for it to work less efficiently, raising your blood sugar levels. In that case, you could be putting yourself at risk for type 2 diabetes and heart disease.

Your Kidneys on Sugar

If you already have diabetes, too much sugar can lead to kidney damage. Your kidneys are essential for filtering the blood in your body. Once blood sugar levels reach a certain point, the kidneys begin to release sugar into the urine. If not controlled, diabetes can prevent the kidneys from doing their job, resulting in kidney failure.

Your Body Weight on Sugar

Probably one of the most significant wake-up calls for those consuming excessive amounts of sugar is the toll it takes on your weight. We have already discussed how sugar turns into fat to be used as energy later. Picture this; you melt a stick of butter into a large container every day, regardless of the amount you use. The container fits five sticks of butter comfortably without it overflowing. You only use a tablespoon of butter a day, but you still need to keep adding to the container. By the end of day seven, you are overflowing the butter container. There is nowhere else for it to go. Now imagine that this is your body. The skin stretches to accommodate excess fat. That is why obese people have such significant amounts of skin left after they have lost dramatic amounts of weight.

Me on Sugar

I look back now and realize I wasn't quite as happy-go-lucky as I thought I was. As long as I had my "fix," I was pleasant. I wouldn't go as far as to say that I was happy though. I was tolerating life, one sugar high at a time.

I wasn't shy about it either. My moods were more unpredictable than a game of Russian roulette. I found out later that my colleagues prayed they wouldn't be on the receiving end of an outburst. I had outbursts? Where was I when this happened? I was looking for sugar and until I found some form of it I was walking in a blind rage.

I have always been a relatively healthy person. No matter where my weight was, my bloodwork always came back impeccable. I don't know if you have ever put on a drastic amount of weight during your lifetime. I did, but I was in denial.

I could look in the mirror and despite my pants not fitting or my shirt being too tight, I still saw the old me. Those items just shrunk in the dryer, right? But they hadn't and once I began seeing what sugar really was doing to my life, it became more apparent that I was trying to live in a fantasy.

Five Serious Diseases That May Be Linked to Sugar

Studies have taken place all over the world regarding how sugar can affect the body. With that said, there have been some pretty thought-provoking links made between disease and sugar intake. I would not have thought that a link existed to some of these, but the more research is done, the more patterns are taking shape. Hello? Are you listening to your body? I wasn't, which is why I believe in doing a sugar detox – jumpstarting the way you can change your body's future.

Cancer

I want to start by giving you some startling statistics. America's National Center for Biotechnology Information did a study on people who at a diet with a high glycemic load (aka lots of glucose/sugar), and they found that the risk of developing prostate cancer was increased by 30%, rectal cancer by 44%, and pancreatic cancer by 41%. I'm not a doctor, nor do I play one on tv, but I have watched enough medical shows to know that pancreatic cancer does not have a very high success rate. Your pancreas creates insulin to help level out your blood sugar. If something goes wrong, you are looking at a minimum of becoming a type 2 diabetic.

Think about this: A study was published in the *Journal of Clinical Investigation*, which points to sugar as a fuel source for existing cancers and the primary factor of initiating cancerous characteristics in healthy cells.

Obesity

Fructose is the largest culprit for weight gain, often investigated because of its counterpart high fructose corn syrup. You have heard the commercials and ads, "contains no high fructose corn syrup," why is that? Studies showed us that excessive amounts of high fructose corn syrup are not healthy. The body has no use for it, it can't do anything with it, and if the liver becomes overloaded, it turns into fat.

The link between obesity and fructose also comes from the study of leptin. Leptin is what is secreted by fat cells to say, "Hey! We are full down here. No more energy storage is needed!" But do we listen? Not really, which is why we end up eating that extra slice of cake or candy bar at odd hours.

Cardiovascular Disease

Sugar is one of the leading indirect causes of cardiovascular disease. Yes, you read that right, indirect causes. It isn't fair to say that sugar itself causes the heart to have problems because it isn't. Sugar is merely the start of the entire process.

When you consume a lot of sugar, it raises your blood sugar levels. In a natural response, the body produces insulin to help reduce the amount of sugar in your blood. The higher your insulin levels are, the higher the risk of inflammation caused to your cardiovascular system.

So the cardiovascular disease is caused by the inflammation caused by the high insulin levels that the pancreas releases to help reduce the amount of sugar in your blood after consuming it. Think of it as a cause and effect situation with the body – the sugar starts a chain reaction that then leads to the disease.

Diabetes

Diabetes is more than just a disease that is associated with high blood sugar levels. There is a significant difference between type 1 and type 2 diabetes. Type 1 is when the body fails to create the insulin needed naturally. Type 1 diabetes is not due to consuming too much sugar.

Type 2 diabetes is associated with obesity, which can be correlated to the overconsumption of sugar, carbohydrates, etc. In some cases, simply losing weight can help reduce or eliminate type 2 diabetes. The insulin resistance caused by higher blood sugar levels can cause more than just weight or pancreatic problems.

People with diabetes who do not take care of themselves or their sugar problems could end up with neuropathy (painful nerve disorder), circulation problems that ultimately can cause amputation, and other life-threatening diseases.

Liver Disease

Liver disease is not a hot item in medical news. Many people don't even realize the problems caused within the liver by excessive amounts of sugar. Sadly, people here cirrhosis and automatically assume alcoholism. That isn't always the case, though.

Fatty liver disease happens when too much sugar is processed through the liver. It turns into fat because it has nowhere else to go. Extensive damage to the liver can lead to scarring. Scarring is what ultimately leads to cirrhosis because the blood supply is cut off from the organ.

I Didn't Know I Was Putting My Life in Danger

Genetics plays a role in a lot of the diseases we can develop during our lifetime. Your mom and dad were obese so the chances of you being obese are even higher. The maternal side of your family had heart problems, making you prone to developing them. You probably know in the back of your mind that these problems exist in your family, but you have the "it can't happen to me" attitude. I know I sure did.

Knowing what I knew about these health problems, what did I do? I poured granulated sugar down my throat (not literally, but I might as well have). When I decided that enough was enough and I was going to make changes in my life, I began finding out just how much my genetics and the problems sugar could have on my body.

I already knew that my weight was becoming an issue, I was out of breath putting my socks and shoes on. So, I knew I was going to be working on that. I just didn't realize it was all the sugar that caused a lot of my problem.

You are probably reading this and thinking that I am a sugar hater. I don't hate sugar, in fact, I was in a passionate relationship with sugar. I LOVE SUGAR. But there will come a time in your life that you realize some relationships are toxic and you must move forward.

Was one more candy bar worth the potential heart attack?

Proof You Are Addicted to Sweetness

Now that you have the sugary background, history, and potential disease factors, it's time to talk about your addiction. If you have made it to this point of the book, it's because you at least suspect that you have a dependency on sugar – you wouldn't be reading this if you didn't.

I want to help you put your doubt aside, and be able to face the sugary demon that is controlling your life. I had to have a serious wake-up call, and now it is time for yours. Here is an interactive test that you can take. Don't fret. It's not graded, and there is no judgment when you reach the realization that maybe you are a sugar addict.

The test is made of 12 true and false statements, so just be honest. You can grab a scrap piece of paper and jot down your answers, and we will discuss the scoring at the end.

Statement	True	False
1. I don't eat any refined sugar on a daily basis		
2. I can go more than one day without eating something that contains sugar		
3. I don't get cravings for sugar, chocolate, coffee, alcohol, or peanut butter		
4. I have never hidden sweet treats around the house so that I		

can eat them later		
5. I can stop eating candy or other baked goods after one		
6. I often run out of sugary items around the house without the urge to get more		
7. I can keep sweet treats in the house without eating them		
8. I can go at least three hours without eating and experiencing shakiness, tiredness, or mood swings		
9. I don't have the urge to eat something sweet after meals		
10. My breakfast rarely consists of sweets like coffee, donuts, or sweet rolls		
11. I can go for more than one hour after waking up without the urge to eat		
12. I don't drink soda or other beverages filled with sugar		

Before we get into the grading, I want to clarify a couple of items. When asked about coffee, it doesn't mean black coffee. It means sugar, cream, or flavored creamer filled cups of sugary caffeine. Also, number four might not be logical if you have kids. How many of us have never hidden candy from our kids? If you said no, you are definitely not telling the truth...it isn't our fault if we don't want to share (it's an addiction).

Now for the grading:

- If you answered four or more of these questions FALSE, you might want to reach out for help with releasing yourself from sugar addiction.
- If you answered between one and three of these questions FALSE, you might be at risk of developing an addiction to sugar later.
- If you didn't answer any of the questions FALSE, you don't have a sugar addiction (or you lied....)

You May Be A Sugar Addict If...

Sugar addiction can affect us in many different forms, but for the most part, we showcase some classic addiction symptoms. From secret candy stashes to mood swings (hangry), each of these symptoms can help you get on the right path to sugar independence. I want to explore some of the common telltale signs that you may suffer from sugar addiction.

You may be a sugar addict if...

You Try To Hide Your Sugary Habit

Some people with sugar addiction may recognize that they have a problem. Instead of finding ways to work through the problem, they choose to keep it out of sight. Out of sight, out of mind – right? WRONG! You are doing a disservice to yourself and everyone around you.

You can make all the excuses you want for why you do what you do, but who are you hurting at the end of the day? If you have to hide that you are eating an entire box of snack cakes for fear of being told you have a problem, you already know you have a problem. The next step is just finding ways to get over it.

Your Cravings Become Hard to Satisfy

Any time addiction is involved, the body's tolerance can change over time. This theory applies to sugar, drugs, alcohol, etc. When it comes to being a sugar addict, your body will crave more and more over time. When one candy bar might have calmed the midafternoon hunger, now it takes two, three, four, or more. The worse the addiction and the cravings, the more likely you are to begin hiding it.

You Eat Sugary Treats Even When You Aren't Hungry

There is a difference between being addicted to food and being addicted to sugar. Many people who don't know squat about addiction will assume that overeating sugary treats are nothing more than a food addiction. These people aren't right, but they aren't wrong, either. Sugar addicts stick to sugary foods whether they are hungry or not, and they may even turn to it as a comfort. Someone who is addicted to food, in general, doesn't stop at sugary treats. They will eat anything they can get their hands on to satisfy their need for emotional comfort. It doesn't matter if you are addicted to food or sugar. In both scenarios, you are often not hungry when you overindulge in your vice.

You Have Constant Cravings

I'm not referring to the song by K.D. Lang when I say constant craving. I'm talking about your body thinking that it needs the sugar. Anytime your blood sugar reaches a "low" level, your mind is automatically going to tell you it needs sugar to get back to the level it was at before the crash. Since you don't like how you feel, you will give in – every time.

You Crave Other Foods

The body is a unique organism. When it lacks something, it will give you the signals relaying that message. For example, have you ever heard of someone who had low levels of potassium craving a banana? The body was saying, "I need potassium, feed me a banana."

The same applies when you fill your body with only added sugar. You miss out on the other nutrients your body needs to function. You may find that your body begins sending you messages in the form of cravings for things like salty foods, starches, or meats. Your body is telling you that it needs more substance to its diet. Added sugars have ZERO nutritional value, which means they are not sustaining your life force at all.

You Try To Kick The Habit, But The Withdrawal Is Too Much

One of the biggest reasons an addict turns back to their vice is that being without it is too hard. This principle can be applied to any addiction. Drug addicts often find themselves hooked on a new drug trying to come off another because they need to get rid of the withdrawal symptoms. Sugar is the same way. If you have been addicted to sugar for a long time, your body will undergo physical changes that may seem too much to handle. You generally "fall off the wagon" and eat sugar to stop those symptoms in those instances.

Sugar Provides You With Emotional Support

In general, addiction often starts because a dependency is formed to help someone cope with some kind of stressor. Your significant other broke up with you? Have a cupcake (or a dozen). You didn't get that promotion at work? Eat a pint of ice cream.

We turn to sugar as a way to handle the stressors in our lives. As an addict, I know all too much that sugar can get you through some of the stickiest situations, no pun intended. Common stressors that people use sugar to solve are anxiety, depression, boredom, and other mental or physical issues.

Despite The Consequences, You Engage Anyway

When you are an addict, the dangers don't apply to you. In your mind, you are invincible, and there is no way you could end up obese, with cancer, diabetes, or cardiovascular disease. With this mindset, you play a Russian roulette game, not sure when your time will be up.

You Make A Point To Get Sugar

Late-night trips to the gas station or 24-hour grocery store to buy candy, cakes, or ice cream can be a sign of your addiction to sugar. Unless you are pregnant and getting cravings for peanut butter and pickle ice cream sandwiches, there probably isn't any reason for you to jump out of bed at midnight to get a sweet treat. This behavior can be a sign of a problem.

You Feel Intense Guilt About Eating Sugar

Here is the scenario:

You eat a ton of sugar. I mean an entire bag of miniature candy bars or a half-gallon of ice cream, whatever the sugary sweetness is, you eat it. After you finish it, you begin to feel guilty about it.

Your guilt brings up feelings that make you uncomfortable, so in your quest for comfort, you seek out sugar. The circle of events, in this case, is never-ending. It will always be the same pattern unless you break the cycle.

My Toxic Relationship with Mr. Ose

I get that this sounds like the byline for a cheesy talk show or a made-for-tv movie, but it really was a toxic relationship. Let's look at all the factors:

- **I tried to hide my habit** – despite my roller coaster of breakups and getting back together, Mr. Ose is not exactly a fan favorite of everyone around me. To stop listening to all the "advice" everyone had for me, I had to hide his existence. For all anyone knew, we were on a strictly platonic level.
- **My cravings became hard to satisfy** – The more our relationship blossomed the more of the danger I craved with Mr. Ose. He knew how to show a girl a good time, and the higher he took me, the higher I wanted to go. There was something about tall, dark, and deadly that I couldn't get enough of.
- **I saw Mr. Ose even when I didn't need to** – I found myself making it necessary to call on Mr. Ose, even when we were apart. I always crossed paths, even if it meant I had to go out of my way.
- **He was all I could think about** – When I woke up in the morning, I craved Mr. Ose. When I had lunch, I craved Mr. Ose. Even at dinner and before bed, Mr. Ose was the only thing on my mind. There were even times in the middle of the night I would wake up with him on my mind, keeping me from a restful sleep.
- **Despite our relationship, sometimes it wasn't enough** – Despite the feelings I had for Mr. Ose, there would be times when I would think of other past relationships. Sometimes I would find myself

dreaming of the days when Mr. Natrium would take me for walks on the beach to take in the salty air or we would share a bag of chips in the park.

- **I knew he was bad, but the feelings were too much** – I tried to leave the toxic relationship with Mr. Ose before, but the feelings that came when we were apart were too much for me to handle. I physically needed him, so I would run back every time.
- **I needed his emotional support** – Despite his toxicity in my life, Mr. Ose was my emotional support. He was the only one who understood when I was sad, depressed, or just bored with life.
- **I knew the dangers, but I kept going back** – I knew how dangerous Mr. Ose could be in my life. I knew that at any moment he could kill me – in broad daylight or in my sleep. Something about the danger kept drawing me in.
- **I made a point to see him** – It didn't matter what time of day it was, when I wanted Mr. Ose, I would find a way. I would drive across town to bump into him at his favorite ice cream place or I would follow him to the grocery just to have an encounter in the parking lot. There was nothing I wouldn't do to be near him.
- **At the end of the day, all I felt was guilt** – Even knowing everything I knew and feeling everything I felt with Mr. Ose, there would come a time when he wasn't around and guilt would move in. The shame I felt for sneaking around and putting my life at risk would flood me. Then I would need his emotional support all over again.

Sounds like a daytime soap opera up for some Daytime Emmy Awards, right? I wish it was that easy. Watching the life of someone else caught in a toxic relationship going through the motions until the villain is killed in a tragic car accident. Then a season later you find out that he was really a twin and the new doctor in town is really his brother Mr. Rose and now you are in the same situation with an equally handsome life wrecking entity.

Luckily, I was able to escape and start new. We still see each other in passing, but I found out just how much better off I was once I let Mr. Ose go.

Chapter Four: The Great Sugar Exodus

Exodus (noun) ex-o-dus: *a mass departure*

Detox (verb) de-tox: *a program or facility for assisting a person undergoing detoxification from an intoxicating or addictive substance*

Deciding that you no longer want to be addicted to sugar can be a difficult decision to make. The word "detox" sounds worse than it is. It is always associated with drug addicts going through withdrawal symptoms, often depicted on the television as some intense and gruesome experience. Is sugar detox easy? No, ridding your life of something that controls you is never easy, especially if you have an addiction.

There is a right and wrong way of doing a sugar detox, which will come along in a later chapter, but for now, I want to emphasize that the process is worth it in the end. I want to take some time to dissect what happens when sugar leaves your body after holding it hostage for a long time. Any time you give up something your body has become dependent upon, you may experience some form of withdrawal. Some symptoms may be more intense than others, but being prepared for them can make the difference between failure and success.

The Effects of Giving Up Sugar

Sugar withdrawal occurs when your body no longer receives the amount of sugar it is used to receiving regularly. When the sugar is no longer being introduced to the body, the body will experience many symptoms. These symptoms manifest mentally, physically, and emotionally.

Why does this happen? Sugar triggers dopamine in the brain – the "happy" hormone. The more you introduce, the more your body becomes dependent on the euphoric feeling. Take away the euphoria, and the body has to learn how to cope without it. Think of it as your body revolting or protesting the lack of sugar you are consuming.

Like giving up any addiction, the severity of the withdrawal will vary from person to person. For me, I wasn't the most pleasant person to be around. I could flip my switch in a matter of seconds, going from anger to weeping all because I saw a candy bar commercial. I didn't want to feel like this, but my body's changes didn't leave me much choice.

After making it through that initial withdrawal period, I will say I felt better and more alive. You will feel the same way, too.

Feelings of Fatigue and Weakness

One of the first withdrawal symptoms that will present itself is fatigue. Shortly after, muscle weakness may or may not join the party. Why do you feel tired when you give up sugar? I know that I said I felt better and more alive, but that comes with more than just a few days of being free from the sugar.

Take a minute to think about what we have talked about, thus far, and how sugar changes your body. Here is a simple equation to illustrate:

Mid-Day Slump + Sugar = Sugar Rush aka Increased Energy

Now, take sugar out of the equation. What are you left with?

Mid-Day Slump + No Sugar = Mid-Day Slump aka Fatigue

Depending on how long you have been using sugar to keep you going, you could experience extreme fatigue. Your body has to recuperate from running on sugar, which is where some muscle weakness can come from. Your body isn't used to not having that extra kickstart. The lower blood sugar levels play a role, but once you get your body regulated, you will see an increase in natural energy, and your strength will return.

Increased and Extreme Cravings

I never said that the process of relieving your body from sugar addiction would be easy. One of the most challenging withdrawal symptoms to deal with is more psychological than physical. Your brain will try everything it can to get its increase in dopamine, including making you think that you have to have it to make it through the day. Ignoring this is easier said than done, but it is possible.

Cravings are a sign of addiction and withdrawal. You can assume that if you haven't had a sugary treat in over 12 hours, your craving is because your body is withdrawing, not because you really need it or want it.

These cravings can be intense. In fact, some cravings are so intense your mouth waters, and you can taste and smell what your brain wants you to. This is what makes it so easy to give up and eat some sugar. That is why when we talk about the method of sugar detox I recommend, it won't be a cold-turkey situation.

Confusion

As the blood sugar in the body lowers, you may experience some confusion. It isn't anything to worry about. It is more of a nuisance than anything. Your brain is looking for its energy fix, and when you don't supply it, the brain deprives you of feeling normal. Confusion is something that can occur in any kind of withdrawal from a substance, including sugar.

Headaches

Headaches are often the body's way of signaling that something is wrong. In addictions like sugar and even caffeine, the brain is being deprived of the extra dopamine or energy rush it craves. It isn't like you can send your brain an email that lays out the entire detox plan in preparation. It only goes through the motions until you give it a new routine. You have to implement the routine for the brain to succumb to it.

For the most part, you will only struggle with the withdrawal headaches for a day or two. You can manage these headaches by using yoga or other calming types of workout. If you experience severe headaches and other neurological problems when reducing or cutting out sugar, you should seek advice from your physician as these could be signs of another underlying condition.

Changes in Behavior

Behavioral changes are often seen in people who are overcoming addiction. You have heard the term "hangry," which is no joke. If your body is hungry, but you aren't giving it what it really wants, you can almost guarantee that your mood is not going to be pleasant. Think of this as a subconscious action, like speaking louder than you intended because you have headphones in your ears. It isn't something you mean to do. Your body just does it as compensation.

Once your brain realizes that you are giving it what it needs instead of what it wants, this symptom should ease up some. This isn't the only behavioral change you may experience, though. Your emotions will likely be questionable for a little while. As your brain and body learn how to adjust and respond to the new chemical balance without the increased dopamine, it will get easier.

Trouble Sleeping

Your body rejuvenates when it sleeps. Think of it as a reset for your mind, body, and soul. When you are sleeping well and get real rest, you find that your energy levels are naturally high, and your health is better. When you are losing sleep, your overall health isn't as good as it could be, which could create other health problems.

Experiencing withdrawal from sugar can cause disturbances in your sleep. This disturbance can take away from the REM cycle of your sleep pattern, which leaves you unrested, possibly cranky, and tired most of the day. Since you are decreasing your sugar levels, you are also decreasing hormones in your body. Usually, these reset within a week or two of cutting out the sugar. If you still experience trouble sleeping, you should discuss your options with your physician.

Depression

You should expect that some level of depression might accompany sugar withdrawal. After all, the dopamine in your brain is not being as stimulated as much as it once was, which means your brain is getting less of that "happy" hormone. Depression can be a severe symptom of withdrawal. If you feel like it is weighing on you and not getting any better, seek medical help. The use of calming and meditative exercising may help you work through your depression. For instance, using structured breathing can help you relax your body and your mind.

The 4-7-8 breathing technique is believed to help with reducing anxiety, helping with relaxation, managing cravings, and controlling or reducing anger response. The technique is easy to do and you don't have to have any "training" for it to be helpful.

1. Breathe in four seconds (or a count of four)

2. Hold the breath for seven seconds (or a count of seven)

3. Exhale for eight seconds (or a count of eight)

You can repeat this as many times as you need to. The idea is to bring a sense of calmness and control over your body.

Unintentional Weight Loss

Weight loss is one of those symptoms you want from sugar withdrawal. When you cut out the additional sugar from your diet, you will likely lose weight because your body is forced to use the excess fat stores for energy. The same can be said when you cut out things like carbohydrates. Your body compensates by using up what is stored within your body, making you lose weight.

Obesity creates serious health risks. Not only does it make the heart work harder, put extra weight on the feet and joints, but it also causes things like high blood pressure in some people. When high levels of sugar are involved, you may even see type 2 diabetes. Reducing or cutting sugar out of your diet can help you begin moving out of the "at-risk" range.

To put it into perspective, obesity has been linked to:

- High blood pressure (hypertension)
- High LDL cholesterol, high levels of triglycerides, and low HDL cholesterol
- Type 2 diabetes
- Coronary heart disease
- Stroke
- Osteoarthritis
- Gallbladder disease
- Sleep apnea
- Cancer
- Lower quality of life
- Mental illnesses
- Body pain
- Difficulty functioning physically
- Mortality

By cutting down on sugar intake or eliminating the added sugars, obesity can be reduced. If for no other reason than to cut down on the risk of developing other serious health problems, you may want to consider cutting out the sugar.

Flu-Like Symptoms (Ketosis)

You have likely heard of the keto diet. Most people have. Part of cutting out sugars means that you are reducing your carbohydrate intake. When you cut out carbohydrates, a process happens within the body, which is called ketosis. Symptoms of ketosis are often compared to the flu. You may get a fever, chills, diarrhea, night sweats, and fatigue. There may be some minor muscle aches and pains associated as well. This occurs because your body uses up the extra fat within the body. You aren't putting any new sugars or carbohydrates in to replace them.

Periods of Lightheadedness

When your blood sugar lowers drastically, you can become lightheaded. In instances where your blood sugar was high for a more extended period of time, and you then stay in a lower range, the symptom may last longer than if it was a temporary drop. Your body will acclimate to the new lower level of blood sugar, and the lightheadedness will subside.

The Five Stages of Sugar Withdrawal

Much like any other significant change in your life, there are stages that you will go through before you reach the "end." For instance, there are stages of working through grief – denial, anger, bargaining, depression, and acceptance. Life-altering changes are something that requires you to mentally, physically, and emotionally work through.

Stage 1: Motivation

When you start something new, the first thing you generally do is find the motivation to do it. You would be surprised at how far a strong will and motivation can carry you when you are determined and set your mind to kicking a habit. I'm not saying that it will always be easy, but for the most part, you will see that your confidence plays a role in your success.

Stage 2: Intense Cravings

We have already covered that your brain is going to work against you before it works with you. The intense cravings you feel in the beginning will be something that will pass. It just takes time. Try to carry your motivation into the second stage of your recovery.

Stage 3: Headaches

Headaches are a common withdrawal symptom, especially when removing sugar from your diet. The headaches typically begin shortly after the cravings start. Still, within a day or two, you should notice that these begin to ease up.

Once you find yourself without the headaches, pat yourself on the back because you are halfway there.

Stage 4: Aches, Pains, and Other Symptoms

This stage begins shortly after the headaches subside and can instill a bit of doubt in your mind. Don't give up, because even though you may feel like you are at your worst right now, the relief is right on the horizon. Stage four is where the onset of depression can set in, so make sure you are doing mental checks with yourself and seeking assistance from medical professionals if you need it.

Stage 5: Symptom Resolution

The struggle has been real, and you can acknowledge that. Stage five is where the real healing begins, though. You have made it through all the stages and went through all of the withdrawal symptoms. That was only the beginning of your journey. Now you have to come up with the plan going forward. You will want to develop a plan to keep your sugar addiction at bay and continue to live your new healthier lifestyle.

How the Withdrawal Affected Me

You wake up one morning, feeling really good. You didn't expect it. For lack of better words you just went through hell and you didn't think you would get past it. At least that is how it was for me. Let's talk about my journey through the abyss and back to solid ground.

Stage 1: Motivation – I started off motivated about the entire thing. I was my own cheerleader, I wasn't going to let anything get me down – no matter what! I assumed that the amount of confidence I had in the beginning would be enough to carry from start to finish. Little did I know it was going to be a lot harder than that. You know what they say about good intentions...

Stage 2: Intense Cravings – Cravings are a lot harder on the body than anyone will tell you. I think if I could have chewed off my arm to get a piece of cake I probably would have. It starts as a thought in the back of your head, only to creep to the front slowly. What's worse is if you see someone else eating sugary treats. I swear I only drooled once lusting after someone's ice cream cone.

Stage 3: Headaches – So I felt like my head had been beaten with 20 sledgehammers at the same time. Okay, maybe I'm exaggerating a bit but it was definitely no less than 15. If you have ever given up caffeine it is a lot like that. I didn't want to think or move because the threat of my head exploding seemed like a sure thing.

Stage 4: Aches, pains, and other symptoms – As my headache seemed to be going away, my body felt like it had taken a beating. Kind of like the aches you get when you have the flu. I didn't want to get out of bed, but I knew I had to. I knew that I wasn't letting my body throw this fit and win.

Stage 5: Symptoms resolve – I woke up one morning, and nothing hurt. I thought for sure that there was something lurking behind my bedroom door, in the closet, or would attack me as soon as I put my foot on the floor – nothing! I didn't believe it at first, to be honest. I had just been through some of the more painful moments in my life, and all because I chose snack cakes over salads.

The experience will be different for everyone. You might feel nauseous, you may get lucky and not have headaches, or who knows, our bodies are truly tricky things. My only hope is that you can make it through like I did. It was definitely worth it.

Overcoming A Sugar Addiction

As I said, the stages of sugar withdrawal are only the beginning of the journey. Once you make it through all the withdrawal symptoms and are ready to start fresh, you have to develop a plan to move past the old addiction and live your new life. It's hard to do, and I won't lie to you. I struggled at first, and I struggle more on some days than I do on others. That is why the plan going forward is critical to your recovery.

Educate Yourself

To completely change your diet means learning what contains sugar and what doesn't. You don't have to completely eliminate all sugar from your diet, which would be next to impossible. Be mindful of sugar. Learn what has natural sugar, added sugar, and artificial sugars. Use this as a guide to creating your diet plan. Using a plan can make you more successful than just winging it.

Make yourself a shopping list. Go through your cabinets and throw out all the temptations that may be lurking within them. You will find a recipe, snack, and alternative food guide in chapter seven, which will make replacing your cabinets that much easier.

I found that making my meal plans a week at a time and only grocery shopping for those items reduced the risk of me slipping back into sugary temptation. Don't worry. I'll give you examples of this, too. I feel like having a plan that facilitates your recovery from sugar addiction is the means by which you can be successful. You are reading this because you want to make a change, and you aren't alone!

Be Realistic With Your Goals

To carry your motivation all the way through, you have to be realistic with the goals you set. You can't honestly think that you will kick a sugar addiction, or any other addiction for that matter, in a week. That is not realistic, nor is it logical. You have to accept that overcoming an addiction, even to sugar, will be something that you have to work at every day from here on out.

Without realistic goals, it is easy for you to give up or just go back to the way it was before. That is why I cannot stress to you enough that being realistic is the key to overcoming. When those cravings hit you, look to alternatives. I always danced or exercised, trying to get my mind off of eating something sweet.

Look For Healthy Alternatives

I get it, healthy alternatives aren't always the most luxurious, and they sure don't taste like a donut drizzled in glaze. Sacrifices have to be made if you want to be healthier and free yourself from the hold sugar can place on your life.

Look to natural fruits and vegetables to fend off your sweet tooth. Although they do have natural sugars in them, they also provide fiber and water, which added sugars do not. There have to be compromises made to achieve your goals.

Turn to Protein

If you want to cut the sugar out of your diet more for weight loss and health, turning to proteins can help satisfy your hunger. By swapping out sugars and some carbohydrates for protein, you can feel full longer and aid in your weight loss journey.

Another plus to adding more protein to your diet is the uncanny ability it has to help fight off sugar cravings. By helping to fight these sugar cravings, it can also help your body fight off the blood sugar fluctuations you may encounter as a result of changing your diet.

In case you had never heard the term, ghrelin is the hormone that controls hunger. This sneaky little hormone is what tells your brain when it is time to eat—the more protein in your diet, the less ghrelin that will be floating around in your system.

Don't Give Up

If you have ever tried to lose weight, change your diet, eliminate sugar, or even just try to drink more water, you will learn quickly that you will fail. I'm not trying to discourage you. I'm trying to do the opposite. I want you to know that if you don't succeed the first time, try again. There is nothing in the "rule book" that says you can't have more than one try at this.

The next section in this chapter will cover the physical changes your body will endure when you reduce or eliminate the added sugars from your diet. I think that understanding your sugar addiction, the withdrawal from sugar, and how your body changes are the foundation that will prepare you for a sugar detox diet.

When I began my journey, I didn't have a guide. I did some research and honestly just went with the changes as they came. That was my motivation to share my story – to give you a realistic view of what sugar detox is and how it can change your life. I won't sugarcoat it (again with the puns). The journey you will embark on won't be easy. But if you trust me and don't give up, you can change your life for the better.

Exodus Invoked Changes – How Your Body Will Change

Kicking a sugar habit is hard. Even with those who have the strongest of wills, sugar withdrawal can create quite a challenge. Added sugar is where a lot of the problem lies. Foods that have natural sugars are metabolized differently. Even just reducing the amount of added sugar you eat can cause your body to change.

What happens when you remove sugar from your diet? You begin to experience changes – changes that come once you reduce the sweetness in your life.

Younger Looking Skin

Part of eating too much sugar is the amount of sugar that ends up in your bloodstream. Studies suggest that having a high blood sugar level sets up glycation. Glycation is the process that can hinder your body's repair of the skin's collagen. Collagen is what gives our skin the plump and natural glow.

A diet heavy in sweet treats can lead to reduced skin elasticity and premature wrinkles. Luckily, research has shown that lowing the amount of sugar in your diet can help lessen the sagging and other visible signs of aging. So the next time you grab that pint of ice cream, ask yourself if it's really worth the extra wrinkles.

Tap Into Lasting Energy

Added sugars are nothing more than simple carbohydrates. These simple carbohydrates get broken down and enter the bloodstream quickly, supplying you with that energy rush. It is a roller coaster, though, replenishing these simple carbohydrates to keep the ride going. When you reduce or eliminate your added sugar intake, your body will go through an energy change.

When you replace the simple carbohydrates with protein or healthy fats, they supply the body with a steadier supply of energy that lasts longer. The release of endorphins during exercise works the same way. Instead of filling your body with added sugars, you can provide it more sustainable energy, avoiding the dreaded sugar crash.

Reduce the Risk of Serious Health Problems

Diets heavy in added sugar can pose a risk to your health. Sugar is like a secret spy, playing different roles in the life of the inhabitants that it secretly stalks. In some, it might show up and facilitate obesity, others high blood pressure, and a multitude of other underlying problems that lead to bigger health scares.

Making the change to detox and change your sugary lifestyle can help with these underlying factors that cause so many other health risks. Heart disease and type 2 diabetes are real problems among those who live lifestyles heavy in added sugar. These are often exasperated by obesity, which can be linked to an overabundance of sugar.

Doing This Now Pays Big in the Long Run

You may not see any real reason to change your lifestyle right away. If you aren't showing signs of obesity, high blood pressure, heart disease, or type 2 diabetes, you may think you have time. But do you have time?

Changing your lifestyle now will greatly benefit your life and your body down the road. Don't get caught ten yea rs from now, wishing that you had listened to me. Try doing the 40-day sugar detox plan and see how much better you feel after you complete it. You might be surprised at just how crummy you felt eating all that sugar, and you didn't even know it!

It Takes Time

We all bounce back at different rates. I didn't wake up to luxuriously flawless skin the day after I gave up sugar. In fact, I never really had poor skin so, I can't attest to how that works. I will say, research says I should not have to worry about premature wrinkles though.

The real win was when I didn't have to worry about my energy levels anymore. I used sugar as a crutch for so long to give me the extra boost that I needed. Those first days were the hardest, trying to go without the sugar and feeling like I was operating on empty all the time. I did learn that the stronger my will got, the more my body seemed to recover. There came a day when I didn't notice sluggishness. That was my tipping point. It was like I got over that hump it was smooth sailing, my body was more naturally energized.

I know I made the right decision because the health risks were real. I was at risk for serious health issues before adding sugar into the equation, after sugar it seems like my future was almost guaranteed. I didn't want to see it at first, nobody does. I was in the habit of doing the wrong things for my body because they felt better than doing the good.

I realized that I could change my fate though, and that when it was all said and done, I would feel good too.

Chapter Five: Detox to Break the Chains of Sugar Addiction

Once you are ready to take on your sugar addiction, you can begin the preparation period for your 40-day detox plan. Chapter six will take you on a more in-depth journey of the detox plan and process, but what I want to focus on right now is you. You have to be prepared to do this – say it out loud, I CAN DO THIS!

Up to this point, maybe you have been skeptical about the message that I am trying to convey with this book. I don't blame you – who am I to tell you about your addiction, right?

AN ADDICT KNOWS AN ADDICT

I know what you are thinking, "did she really just say that?" Yes, eager patron reading this book, I did, and I'm not ashamed to admit it. You have to stop letting yourself feel like sugar isn't an addiction because it is sugar. If you want to be able to break the chains it holds on your life, you have to accept that sugar is your drug, and you are an addict.

What makes me qualified to tell you how to approach your problem? I don't hold a Ph.D. in Nutrition, nor do I have a Masters in Psychology – what I do have is the experience of being in your shoes, doubting these very words.

I am a recovering sugar addict. That is why I am qualified to share my story and lead you out of the darkness and into the light!

Preparing for the Sugar Detox

I have said it already, and I'll probably say it half a dozen more times before you reach the end of the book – PREPARATION AND ORGANIZATION ARE KEY!

I'm really not trying to sound like a broken record. Still, there will come a time in the upcoming weeks where you will find yourself doubting everything I said to you, and you will doubt yourself. I doubted myself at the very beginning, but I didn't get to a point where I wanted to throw in the towel until somewhere around day 30.

That's right, and I almost threw in the towel ten days shy of reaching my goal – but I didn't. You have to see it as a blessing, the emotions that you will go through. The only way you can do that is to prepare for the worst and hope for the best.

Day 30 was one of those days that you never want to relive. Everything went wrong, and I was just going through a lot. I went out with some friends, and they were all eating whatever they wanted, and there I sat, drooling over the hot fudge sundaes. Even though they meant well, each of them only asked me about a gazillion times if I wanted one or wanted to share.

"Come on, just take one bite!"

One bite. I could handle one bite, right? I mean, no one would know that I did it, and I don't have anyone to answer to.

What is the cost of one bite? The last 29 days of strength and motivation down the drain because of one bite of hot fudge sundae. Do you want to start back at day one?

A little insight into the inner workings of my brain right there – good cop/bad cop. I didn't do it. I could have. There wasn't anyone making me give up the added sugar except for myself. I had to be accountable for my actions, though. It was important to me to see this thing through.

With that said, no one will judge you if you fall off the wagon for a minute. Hold yourself accountable and start over again. You will be your worst enemy when it comes to this part. Don't sweat it, and don't let temptation rock the boat.

What does preparation look like?

- Pick a date to start your detox plan. Be realistic with this. Tomorrow or the day after is not feasible so try to get a date that is at least a week in the future.
- Use this week to prepare your house for a lifestyle change. I don't call it a diet because you might choose to continue with this after the 40 days, making it a lifestyle change.
- Create sections of the pantry and refrigerator that are only yours. Move anything from that area that will not be conducive to the changes you are making.
- Go through and start the menu for the first week of your detox. You may want to do some research on the types of sugar-free snacks that are premade because you may or may not want to cook in the

beginning. Make things that can be done ahead of time. That way, you aren't scrambling last minute to go to the store.

- When possible, use the grocery pick-up feature at your supermarket. How many times have you walked in for one thing and walked out with a cart full of cookies and ice cream?

Find a Support System

Ideally, getting your family on board with the detox would solve a lot of problems. It is understandable, though, if they don't feel the personal motivation to do it. Once they see how much better you feel, they may change the way they feel about it.

Either way, you need to be able to reach out to someone, anyone. Someone who is willing to listen or offer advice is helpful. Even finding social media groups for this purpose can be a great support system. No matter where it comes from, you need positive reinforcement during this time.

Find someone who is willing to make you accountable for your actions. A person who will bust your chops if you backslide and ruin all of your progress. I don't mean that they belittle you, they simply don't take your excuses (because you will have them if you fail).

Restructure Your Reward System

Like a child in school, getting stickers for being good, we like to be rewarded for our accomplishments. How do we normally reward our accomplishments? Yep, with food. When I accomplished something major, I was a pint of ice cream kind of girl. I had to change how I rewarded myself for doing well with my detox program. It really isn't feasible to pop open a pint of ice cream to celebrate being sugar-free.

What is something you want but normally can't justify the purchase? Maybe it is a movie or a novel that was just released, but you don't really have the reason to get it. For example, a new hardback novel just came out that you want to read. The book's price is $30 ($29.99, but what's a penny?). Let's say that during the first 20 days of the detox plan, you have a total of ten goals you meet and achieve. If each of these goals translates to a $4 pint of ice cream, you have $40 additional dollars and can justify the purchase of the book!

Accept That You Might Fail

Not exactly something you want to prepare for, but knowing how you will cope with messing up can be the difference between getting back on the sugar detox wagon and completely giving up. If you can acknowledge that you might fail more than once trying to change your eating habits and sugar intake, you will find that positivity is easier to achieve when it does happen.

Prepare to Put in the Time and Effort

Going through a sugar detox is a lot of work. I'm not going to pretend that it is something that will be easy. You will have days when you are happy, sad, angry, frustrated, and maybe even some days where you don't know how you feel about anything.

You can prepare for those before they happen. Create a happy playlist to get you through the sad. Write yourself a note on a good day to read on a bad day. You will find that in the beginning, the changes will consume your every thought, but this too will pass.

As you advance through the stages and days, you will notice positive changes occurring, probably one of the most remarkable being the increased energy you didn't know existed within yourself.

Do Not Approach This as Easy

I had to start over a couple times, I really don't think it is possible to get it right the first time. I came into it with the attitude that it was going to be an easy thing and we would be on our way to living without sugar. I didn't realize just how much sugar was in my life. I think that was when I realized this wasn't going to be an easy process.

I was going to have to find myself some new coping mechanisms if I was going to make it through.

Exercise Through the Withdrawal

Exercise is one way to work through your withdrawal symptoms. In fact, I recommend using exercise as a way to keep your mind on track during the detox process. I get it. You don't necessarily want to exercise when you are depressed. I promise once you get motivated, the exercise will make all the difference.

Not only can exercise help with depression and anxiety, but it can also help with other physical ailments. For example, those who suffer from high blood pressure, arthritis, and diabetes may benefit from an exercise regimen.

How Does Exercise Help?

Exercising releases endorphins. Endorphins are a "happy hormone." We have talked about how your brain gets a surge of dopamine when you eat sugar. The dopamine affects the brain's reward system and is associated with multiple functions, including, but not limited to, pleasurable sensations, learning, memory, and motor function.

Endorphins are the body's natural pain reliever. The chemical gets released within the body as a result of stress or discomfort. These levels can increase when you partake in rewarding activities, like eating or working out.

When you exercise and create a regimen, you can take your mind off of your worries. It is often called a "runner's high," but it is the release of endorphins that bring a feeling of euphoria. This euphoria can help combat the stress, anxiety, and other symptoms of withdrawal you may encounter during your sugar detox.

Get Your Confidence Back

Exercising makes you feel good about yourself. The first thing we tend to lose when we are going through an emotionally traumatic time, like withdrawal, is our self-confidence. You may think that getting your groove back is impossible, but I'm here to tell you that impossible really means I'M POSSIBLE.

The first rule for exercising – don't set your expectations too high. If you have too high expectations, you can set yourself up for failure, which is something we don't want to do right now. So start simple like a thirty-minute walk each day, anything to be active.

As you reach your goals, you will gain more confidence, allowing you to add a little more to your goals each time. Reward yourself with one of our treats found in the recipes section!

Get More Social

When sugar has been your only friend for a long time, getting out and exercising may open up other opportunities. If you choose to take walks in the park or your neighborhood, you are likely to see other people getting active as well. Even if you only exchange a smile or a "hello," your mood is boosted due to this act.

Healthy Coping Mechanism

For too long, your only method of coping with life has been sugar. When life throws a curveball, you eat a donut. When you get dumped, you eat a pint of ice cream. You feel sluggish, and you reach for a candy bar. These are coping mechanisms, even if you don't realize it.

What can you do to change how you cope with the everyday stressors of life? Exercising is one way to replace those destructive habits with healthy ones. Granted, most likely cannot stop and exercise during the mid-day sugar craving, but there is hope yet. Learning breathing activities can be just as rewarding as a sugar high.

Using the 4-7-8 breathing technique can bring relaxation among those who practice it. It is also great for reducing anxiety. To do this exercise, breathe in for four seconds. Hold this breath for seven seconds. Then exhale for eight seconds. You don't have to sit there and time yourself, just mentally count 4-7-8.

"Exercise" Isn't Always Exercise

The term "exercise" can be used to broadly define anything that describes active movement or stimulation. Using mental exercises can be just as fulfilling as running laps or lifting weights. Even something as little as walking to the copy machine and back can create enough stimulations to help you get over that slump.

Research has shown that getting thirty minutes or more of activity three to five days a week may help with depression or anxiety. If you can't devote that much time at once, breaking it down into smaller increments may be just as beneficial.

How To Get Started Boosting Yourself Through Exercise

Starting and sticking to a new routine can be challenging at first. I'll be the first to tell you that I had to start over a lot when I began this process. Finding a buddy to do this with can help, but if you don't have someone who wants to give up sugar with you, you can use yourself as motivation. There are things that you can do to help yourself through this process.

Figure out what you enjoy doing – We all get caught up in life. I know I forgot what those things were that gave me joy before I filled the void with sugar. The busier I got, the less often I listened to the things I needed, the more I shoved sugar in my face.

It wasn't that I didn't like doing the things I enjoyed. It was just easier to pick ice cream over taking a jog. Figure out what all those things were that you enjoyed doing before life seemed to take over. Was it riding a bike? Going for a walk?

Set reasonable goals for yourself – You should start by making your goals for being active reasonable. Don't set out thinking that you can do everything all at once. Come up with a plan that starts light. The more you try to take on at once, the more overwhelmed you may feel. The more overwhelmed you feel, the more likely you are to give up.

Don't make it a chore — Making exercising another mandatory thing in your life can make you not want to do it. How often do you not want to do the dishes and let them pile up? You know you have to do them, but you don't want to. Exercising is the same way. You know you should do it, but the idea isn't all that appealing. Make it fun — make it a reward!

Look at the barriers that may exist — Is there something that could set you back? Sometimes our mind plays tricks on us and makes us way too self-conscious about exercising in public. The barrier created might be fixed by starting your routine at home. Are you worried that time might be a factor? You can break up the amount of time you want to exercise into several parts of your day. Nothing says that it has to be all at once. For most of the barriers, you may be able to find a solution that can help you overcome the obstacle.

It is okay to have setbacks — You have to give yourself credit, even for the little accomplishments. Only acknowledging the setbacks can make the process have a negative connotation, which can be discouraging.

Honesty is the Best Policy - *Author Confession*

Before we get into exercises, I have to be honest with you. I came into exercise with little knowledge of anything. I've never been an active person, but I knew I needed a distraction. You do not have to be good at exercise for it to work.

I still try to do yoga, but my body doesn't necessarily agree that it should bend in such ways. Consider me a work in progress in that area. Even though I use exercise as a distraction, it doesn't mean I'm good at it or that I will ever be good at it. I guess what I want you to know is that you don't have to be perfect. You don't even have to be structured if you don't want to be. It took me a long time to not feel weird practicing meditation, and that requires no real physical exertion!

Using Meditation

Meditation has positive effects on the body, even if it wasn't why you were doing it. Studies have found that the relaxation response can have these short-term benefits:

- Lower blood pressure
- Lower heart rate
- Slower respiratory rate
- Lower blood cortisol levels
- Less stress
- Improved blood circulation

- Less perspiration
- Less anxiety
- More feelings of well-being
- Deeper relaxation

Meditation is something that takes practice. You probably won't get it right the first time or the second time, but you can find a way to relax if you keep with it.

The idea is to start simple. Begin with five minutes at a time and work yourself up to longer periods. You can use meditation anytime you need to find a little relief from overwhelming withdrawal symptoms.

Simple Meditation for Beginners

If you are just now starting out, using a beginner's meditation exercise can help you begin practicing. You can use this exercise as a foundation to build upon.

1. Sit or lie on the floor comfortably. Use a pillow, cushion, anything you feel might help make your experience more calming.

2. Close your eyes – some people use refreshing eye masks during this time, but it is not a requirement.

3. Don't try controlling your breath; instead, allow your breath to come and go naturally.

4. Focus your attention on your breath and how your body moves with each inhale and exhale. Observe how your

chest, shoulders, belly, and ribcage all move with it. Focus all your thoughts on only the breath – don't try to control its pace or intensity. If you find your mind wanders off (which it will), bring it back to the breath.

Do this for two or three minutes at first. Try building upon it and focusing longer.

Using Walking Meditation

Since walking is a good way to increase endorphins, walking meditation can help with endorphins and relaxation. Kind of like counting your breath, it's about counting the steps you take – to ten.

1. Begin walking at a natural, slow pace.

2. Make sure you are walking with good posture. Bend your arms at the elbow, bringing your left hand to lay against your diaphragm. Put your right hand in front of it, crossing your thumbs. Your arms should be horizontal with the ground. This stance helps to keep balance and stability while walking.

3. Match each step to your breath. Start out breathing naturally while you walk. Match your breath for your steps. The in-breath is shorter, so it may be fewer steps than the out-breath.

4. Count your steps. On the in-breath count 1-2-3, out-breath 1-2-3-4.

5. Be mindful of the situation. Allow yourself to be fully present at the moment as you count each of the steps.

Focus on the breath and the movement of your legs between each count.

6. Acknowledge anything that arises. As you walk, your focus will be on the walk and the breathing, but other things will make their way into your mind. Don't judge them. Simply acknowledge them and allow them to pass, shifting your observation back to your walking and breathing.

Mindful Body Scan

The mindful body scan takes longer to complete, typically thirty to forty-five minutes. Still, it can be condensed to a shorter version if time does not permit a long session. This exercise allows you to look into yourself and get in touch with what you are truly feeling. It is recommended that you lay down for this exercise, but you can sit if you prefer. All you need is a quiet place where you won't be interrupted.

The best part about this is that there are no right or wrong answers – you just get to be you!

1. From your comfortable position, close your eyes to help your ability to focus.

2. Bring awareness to your body by breathing in and out. Notice the pressure of your body against the seat or the place in which you are lying. There is no time constraint for this. Take as much time as you need to explore how each pressure point feels on the various parts of your body.

3. When you are ready to start, intentionally breathe in. Move your attention to whatever part of the body you wish to investigate. In a full-body scan, it is recommended to start with the head or the feet.

4. Sensations can be anything – buzzing, tingling, tightness, pressure, temperature change, or any other feeling you might notice while you concentrate. You will become more aware in this state, as all your focus is on the one part.

5. Be open and curious about the feelings you are noticing. Investigate as intensely as you possibly can. Chip away at all the layers to get to the root. Once you are ready to move to the next area, allow your focus to drift off and then shift back.

6. The more you practice this, the more you will learn that you can keep your attention from wandering off while you focus. There is no need to force it. You can take your time and go with the flow – wherever it takes you.

7. Whenever you notice your attention wandering, acknowledge it, and gently bring it back. You can do this over the course of your entire body. There is no need to force it, and you can take your time.

8. At the end of your body exploration, take a few moments to feel your body breathing and your breath expanding through your entire body. Move mindfully into this moment.

We can use these methods to create new pathways in the brain. Neuroscience shows that noticing your drifting attention and gently returning it repetitively is how these are formed.

Using Yoga

Yoga can be a great place to start if you want to work with the mind and the body. If you aren't a yogi like me, you can try using some beginner's yoga to get your mind and body ready. The important thing is to listen to your body and adjust the exercises to fit your body and activity level.

The Mountain Pose

The mountain pose is the foundation for all standing poses. This pose gives you a sense of how to ground your feet and feel the earth below you. Don't mistake this pose as "just standing," a lot is going on.

Begin by standing with your feet together. Press down through all ten toes as you spread them open. Actively engage the quadriceps, gaining a feeling up through the knee caps and the inner thighs. Bring the abdomen in with your chest up and the top of your shoulders downward.

You should feel your shoulder blades moving toward one another as you open up your chest. Keep the palms of your hands facing inward toward your body. Imagine that it is a string attaching the crown of your head to the ceiling and breathe deeply through the torso. Hold this for five to eight breaths.

Downward Facing Dog

This position is used in most yoga practices and classes. The exercise stretches and strengthens the entire body.

Get into a position on all fours with your wrists positioned under your shoulders and knees under your hips. Tucking your toes under, bring your hips up and off the floor as you draw back toward your heels.

With your knees slightly bent, keep your hamstrings tight, trying to straighten your legs while moving your hips back. You can then walk forward with your hands to give yourself more length if needed.

Press firmly with your palms, rotating the inside of your elbows toward each other. Hollow the abdominals and engage your legs to stop the torso from moving to the thighs. Hold for five to eight breaths before dropping back down to the starting position.

Plank

The plank teaches balancing on our hands while we use the entire body for support. The plank is a great exercise for strengthening the abdominals and leaning to use the breath to help stay in a challenging pose.

Starting in a position on all fours on the floor, tuck your toes under, lifting your legs off the mat. Slide your heels back enough that you feel you are one straight line of energy from your head through your feet.

Engage the lower abdominal muscles and draw your shoulders back. Pull your ribs together and breathe deep for eight to ten breaths. Return to the natural starting position.

This exercise resembles a push-up without the up and down motion.

The Tree

The tree is a pose that allows for beginners in yoga to work on their focus and gaining clarity. This pose will help you learn to breathe while standing and keeping the body balanced on one foot.

Start with the mountain pose. Bring your right foot up to rest on your inner upper thigh. Press your hands in a prayer position, finding a spot in front of you to focus your gaze on.

Hold and breathe for eight to ten breaths, then switch sides. Be sure not to lean into the standing leg, keeping your abdominal muscles engaged and your shoulders relaxed.

Bridge Pose

The bridge pose is good for the beginner before leaning back bending poses. This pose will stretch the front of the body and strengthen your back.

Begin by laying on your back with your feet flat on the floor, hip-width apart. Press firmly with your feet, lifting your bottom off the mat. Interlace your hands together and press your fists down to the floor as you open up your chest.

Imagine dragging your heels on the mat closer to your shoulders to engage the hamstrings. Hold this for eight to ten breaths, then lower your hips down. Repeat two more times.

Building Your Yoga Sequence

I have given you some very basic beginner's poses for starting out in the yoga world. You aren't likely to find only these positions when you visit a yoga class, but these exercises can help you get started at home. You can make your own yoga sequence that you are comfortable with, here is an example:

1. Start with stretching and breathing. Use meditation techniques to focus on your breath as you are getting your body ready and stretching out your muscles. You should spend at least ten minutes with your breathing and your

stretches – focusing on your hips, waist, back, legs, shoulders, neck, and arms.

2. Begin with the mountain pose. Hold this position for a few minutes, letting the energy flow through your body from the top of your head through the soles of your feet.

3. When you are ready, bring your body down and go into the downward dog. Hold this pose for a few minutes, focusing on your breathing and nothing else around you.

4. Bring your body back up to the mountain pose, allowing your body to rest before transitioning to the next pose.

5. Bring your arms up and your foot to form the tree pose. Hold on the left side for a few minutes (it is okay if you are wobbly at first, balance comes with practice), then switch to the right side and hold for a few minutes.

6. Move into the bridge pose to help stretch the front of the body. Hold this for a few minutes.

7. Transition yourself into the plank position. Hold for a few minutes, paying attention to your breaths.

8. Bring your body to a seated position. Meditate for the last five to ten minutes, feeling the strength as it flows through your body.

As you learn to execute these exercises you will be able to learn some new ones to add to your mix. You can create the yoga sequence that works best for your body.

Strength Training

Strength training tones your muscles, and they bring mental strength and focus as well. Strength training can help benefit the heart, improve balance, strengthen the bones, aid in losing weight, and, most importantly, boost your mood and motivation! I get it. Who wants to sweat?

These types of exercises weren't on my list of things to do. When I was going through the sugar detoxification process, I had a lot of energy from not knowing what to do with myself. It was a good outlet to put my excess energy to good use.

Yoga is considered a strength training exercise, so the plank and bridge are often found on lists of exercises for strength training. There are variations to these exercises, which I will explain in this section.

The Plank – Strength Training Variation

The plank is considered a core exercise, but it can be more than the traditional variation you see in yoga. You can strengthen various areas by focusing on other parts of the body – side plank, leg-lift plank, and forearm plank.

To challenge yourself, you can try any of these:

- **Side plank** — Lie on your side with your knees bent, propping yourself up on your elbow. Raise your hips

119

off the floor, which will straighten out your legs. Hold this for six breaths. Allow yourself to return to the original position, resting for ten seconds. Repeat three to five times.

- **Leg-lift plank** – Start in the traditional plank pose. You can do this with your forearms on the ground or your hands planted on the ground, shoulder-width apart. While breathing, lift one leg off the floor to the hip level, hold for the remaining breaths. Repeat with the other leg. Hold for a count of six to eight breaths, resting for a few seconds in between.
- **Forearm plank** – Much like the traditional plank, only you are resting your weight on your forearms, not your hands. You can do this position in combination with the leg-lift plank as well.

The Bridge – Strength Training Variation

A bridge helps to strengthen the lower half of your body. For the most part, a common bridge is done like the traditional yoga stance, but with the hands flat on the floor. You can make this even more challenging by adding your spin. For example, you can turn your bridge into a leg-lift bridge. The options are endless for customization.

Squats

Squats are a great strength training exercise, but they require you to build up your endurance. You can also create your own variations using free weights and resistance bands.

To properly do a squat, start in a standing position with your feet approximately shoulder-width apart. Keep your arms down at your sides.

Bend your knees and hips, lowering your torso toward the ground. Keep your back straight while doing this.

As you lower your body, lift your arms in front of you so that they are parallel to the ground. Return to the standing position.

Try and repeat in sets of 20, but if you can't do that many at first, just increase as you go forward.

Aerobic Exercises

You may find yourself in the same boat I was in with sugar. I wasn't living my best life, and I was carrying around a little bit of extra padding. Lucky for you, aerobic exercises can help you lose weight. To lose weight, you have to get your heart pumping to burn fat and calories.

Aerobic workouts don't have to be those complicated synchronized exercise programs you see in movies or online. As long as you are active for at least thirty minutes a day, three to five days a week, you are doing enough. You can certainly do more and using these smaller exercises to replace the sugar cravings.

These exercises may seem simple and don't necessarily consume a lot of your time, making some of them perfect for just about any time. Don't laugh at the idea of these because they are going to become your best friend through thick and thin.

Skipping Rope

There isn't a whole lot of instruction that goes into skipping rope. You stand with your feet shoulder-width apart and swing the rope over your head. Doing this for forty-five minutes can burn as many as 450 calories, and it works the muscles in your shoulders, calves, quads, and glutes.

Don't expect to be an all-star athlete skipping a rope thousands of miles an hour (exaggeration – one of the world records is 108 skips in 30 seconds). You can start steady and just build up your endurance if you want to lose weight. I just find doing it for leisure can be fun too.

Jumping Jacks

Jumping jacks work your total body. Stand with your feet together and your hands alongside your thighs. Jump, spreading your feet to the side and reaching your arms above your head. With the next jump, bring your arms back down and your feet back together, all simultaneously. For results, do this for thirty minutes. Since that can seem like a monotonous amount of time to do jumping jacks, break it into three sessions with five-minute breaks between sets.

Stair Training

I recommend doing this where you can use a set of sturdy bleachers. Go up and down a set of stairs for fifteen to twenty minutes and a decent pace. You can work toward building the pace and increasing the speed. If you work in an office, you can do this on your lunch break in the stairwell.

Mountain Climbers

Mountain climbers seem easy at first, but they work on the abs, hips, glutes, and legs. Start in the plank position with your core tight. Bring your right knee up toward the center of your stomach, then quickly switch to the left leg. Start slow and increase gradually. Do one to two sets of eight to ten reps.

Burpees

Burpees are intense – and require a bit of finesse. If you are "graceful" like I am, practice in an area with nothing around you. Stand with your feet shoulder-width apart and get into a squat position. Bending forward, place your palms in front of your feet, stretching out into a plank position. Immediately return to a squat and then back to standing with a jump. Ideally, you should do three to five sets of eight to fifteen reps. Realistically, as someone who ate way too much sugar for a long time, just getting down the basic structure is a workout!

Donkey Kicks

This exercise is easy to accomplish and works on your glutes and hips. Get on all fours with your hands and shoulders aligned, and your knees and hips aligned. Lift your right leg in the air and bring it back down. Do the same with the left. Do three sets of fifteen to twenty repetitions each.

Walking

Walking can seem mundane, but it can do a lot for the body. It can help maintain a healthy weight, strengthen bones, improve balance, improve coordination, and help manage heart disease, type 2 diabetes, and high blood pressure.

Walking can become monotonous though – same path, the same scenery, and the same playlist. How can you change it up? There are different things you can do to entertain yourself, even if you are walking.

You can start by just looking at your surroundings when you go for a walk. Take time to appreciate the nature around you. Listen to the sounds and notice the colors of the world around you.

Try making your walk time an educational time. You can listen to podcasts and learn a new language or listen to an audiobook. Use your walking time as a mentally productive time.

Just Be Active

I can give you a hundred different exercises that will help you preoccupy your time and keep your mind off of your withdrawal symptoms. Some of them may work, others may not. The thing that you have to remember is that being active may be all it takes to create the change in your life. If you like bowling, go bowling. If you like swimming, go swimming. You aren't limited to yoga or meditation. You don't have to only do jumping jacks.

I'm not an exercise expert by any means and I definitely don't necessarily enjoy some of the exercises people do (you will likely never see me running). The point is being active. If you sit still, your body stews over the cravings and the withdrawal and you are likely to give in.

Chapter Six: A 40-Day Sugar Detox Plan

Making the decision to go through a sugar detox program is a huge step at becoming free from sugar. You have struggled with the hold that it has had on your life for so long that you probably are unaware of the detriment it is causing to your body.

If you suffer from sugar addiction, there are three different ways you can approach your situation. The approach you take will be a personal preference. These include cold turkey, incremental, and a hybrid method. For me, a hybrid method worked better than just cutting down or giving it up at the drop of a hat.

No matter which of the three you choose, you need to make sure you have a plan in place. Your plan should be what guides you through the process of the detox. Your plan should be in order before you begin. That way, you aren't scrambling to figure out things last minute.

Cold Turkey Method – Using a cold turkey method can seem a bit drastic (and stressful) if you have been a sugar addict for a long time. You set a date, and on that day, you begin abstaining from the sugar you made the plan for.

Incremental Method – Incremental methods require that you take your plan and spread it out over an extended time frame. During this time, you will cut down your sugar intake a little at a time and work on the behavioral changes that come with it.

Hybrid Method — Take a little bit of this and a little bit of that, and you have the hybrid method. At least that is what I call it. I can be strong-willed, but not where sugar is concerned, so making a plan to go cold turkey would have only made all the areas around me a war zone. The incremental method seems nice in theory, but it left a lot of room for me to slip. I knew if I slipped when I was detoxing, I wouldn't get back on the wagon. (You know a cupcake sounds more luxurious than headaches and depression.)

The hybrid is where my 40-day sugar detox plan came from. There are a lot of different plans on the market today, but none of them really fit me — I had to come up with something that worked and fit my situation. What if it was adaptable? I could help others who want to break free of sugar addiction too.

The Birth of a Plan

I already told you I woke up one morning and I was done. I needed to get rid of the extra sugar in my life. I set out looking for a plan that would work with my life and my personality. I needed to be accountable for my decisions, too, not just follow like a blind sheep.

Low and behold, there wasn't a whole lot out there that piqued my interest. I set out to create something that I thought I might be able to follow. Something that took a pinch of this, a dab of that, and then I mixed it with a whole lot of drive – that is how this 40-day sugar detox plan was born.

The premise of the plan is to break the detox into five stages:

- Stage 1: Days 01-10
- Stage 2: Days 11-20
- Stage 3: Days 21-30
- Stage 4: Days 31-40
- Stage 5: Day 41 and Beyond

I wanted to represent this plan visually, making it easier to see the progress. I didn't stop there. I wanted to give it a little more gusto. I didn't want to do a 40-day plan that I just kept track of on a calendar, marking off the days until I reached the end. Shouldn't it be a beginning instead of an end?

Where should you begin? I began with food and drinks. I didn't automatically cut out all groups with added sugar. I made it a process.

You can use the table below to help you plan your meals for each of the stages. Here is how it works:

- Start by filling in which stage of the detox you are on – 1, 2, 3, 4 (there is not a spot for "beyond")
- In each of the day groups, circle the number of the day. As an example, Stage 1: 1, 2, 3, 4, 5, 6, 7, 8, 9, 10.
- Next, you can start filling in the breakfast for those days, then the lunch, etc.

I have placed the table on its own page so that you can print out the number of copies you need so that you can fill it out. Organization during this process will be your best friend!

Stage ——— Day	Breakfast	Lunch	Dinner	Snack
1 11 21 31				
2 12 22 32				
3 13 23 33				
4 14 24 34				
5 15 25 35				

6				
16				
26				
36				
7				
17				
27				
37				
8				
18				
28				
38				
9				
19				
29				
39				
10				
20				
30				
40				

Making Changes To Reduce Sugar

There are different ways you can change your lifestyle to help facilitate a reduction in sugar. The best way to make these changes is to gradually increase the changes. When the body experiences too much stress at once, you may be more likely to fall off the wagon and back into the arms of added and refined sugar.

Stop Drinking Your Sugar

One of the common ways we intake sugar without fully realizing it is through what we drink. Soda, fruit juice, and other types of drinks are high in sugar content. The best way to eliminate a majority of the sugar is to break up with soda, fruit juice, and other drinks high in added sugar.

Increase the amount of water you drink – the recommendation is 64 ounces per day or more. Water also helps to flush the sugar from your system, as well as any other toxins that might be lingering within your bloodstream. If you are not properly hydrated, you could just be recirculating the toxins within your body.

You can make water fun. Add lemon slices, lime, or cucumber for a flavorful infusion. Despite the natural sugars found in fruits, they are metabolized differently, not hindering the detox. If you want to skip all sugar, you could just opt for the plain water.

What Increasing Protein Can Do During Sugar Detox

In the health world, fats and carbohydrates have their own level of controversy about them that nobody can seem to agree on. The one thing that every healthy eater can agree on is that protein is important. For the most part, our diets include enough protein to prevent a deficiency. Still, the body can do better with a higher intake of protein. Studies have been done and suggest that high-protein diets have major benefits within the body.

Reduce Appetite and Hunger

Studies show that protein is the most filling out of the three macronutrients (fats, carbs, and protein). Protein can reduce the level of your body's hunger hormone, ghrelin. It can also boost the levels of peptide YY, the hormone responsible for making you feel full.

Muscle Mass and Strength

Proteins are the essential building blocks of your muscles. If you plan on increasing your physical activity levels to help with the withdrawal from sugar and the cravings, you are going to need to replenish these proteins. You will likely lose weight when you begin cutting out sugar and exercising. Protein helps you lose fat and not muscle mass.

Bone Health

There was once a myth that suggested that animal proteins were bad for your bones. This myth has since been debunked by studies showing the opposite. Those people who eat higher amounts of protein are more likely to maintain their bone mass as they age. They also have a lower risk of fractures and osteoporosis.

Reduces Cravings and the Need for Late-Night Snacking

Cravings are not the same as feeling hungry. Hunger is your body's request for nutrients. Cravings are your brain's request for a reward. Sugar is what satisfies your brain's reward centers, at least for a short time. Increasing the protein intake can help to reduce or even eliminate the cravings.

Boosts Metabolism and Increases the Burn

Eating high protein can boost metabolism and increase the number of calories you burn. You may not be too concerned with the calories you burn or the weight you lose when you do this sugar detox, and that is okay – I just want to emphasize that protein is going to be an essential part of replenishing your body and fueling it while you cut out the sugar.

Lowers Blood Pressure

High blood pressure causes a majority of strokes, heart attacks, and chronic kidney disease. The higher protein intake has been shown to help lower blood pressure. There were even studies that show protein may reduce bad cholesterol and triglycerides.

Include Healthy High-Fat Foods

I already pointed out that carbohydrates and fats have been labeled as enemies. Since this happened, more sugars, processed foods, and refined carbs entered the scene. Collectively, we have gotten fatter and sicker because of this. Foods that are high in monounsaturated and polyunsaturated fats are good for the body.

- Avocados - most fruits contain carbohydrates, but avocados are loaded with fats. The main fatty acid is oleic acid, a monounsaturated fat.
- Cheese – cheese contains protein, nutrients, and fatty acids, which provide the body with multiple benefits.
- Dark chocolate – as long as the content of cocoa is above 70%, you can be assured that there will be an abundant amount of nutrients, fatty acids, and antioxidants in your chocolate.
- Whole eggs – the yolk of an egg were once considered unhealthy because of the amount of cholesterol that can be found within it. Now studies are showing the contrary to be true. They are loaded

with vitamins and minerals, with the best being omega-3 enriched or pastured.

- Fish – fatty fish like salmon, mackerel, herring, trout, and sardines are rich in heart-healthy omega-3 fatty acids, high in protein, and contain other essential nutrients.
- Nuts – nuts are full of healthy fats and other vitamins and minerals. Studies have shown that people who eat nuts tend to be healthier and have lower risk factors for obesity, type 2 diabetes, and heart disease.
- Chia seeds – not traditionally thought of as fatty food, chia seeds actually have heart-healthy omega-3 fatty acids, including ALA.

Choose Fresh Fruit and Vegetables in a Pinch

Realistically, you can't avoid every tidbit of sugar in every food for the rest of your life. It is not feasible. So if you find yourself at a crossroads with dessert, my recommendation is to choose the fruit. Fruits and vegetables have natural sugars within them, healthier than the excessive amounts of added sugar found in other food items.

When you are starting out with the detox process, you may want to avoid fruits for a limited amount of time to help reset your body. In a healthy and balanced diet, people should be eating two to three servings of fresh fruit a day.

Reach for Healthy Snacks

Cravings are likely to be your biggest enemy during your detox. Giving in to the sugar will only set back your progress and extend the withdrawal time. When you need to snack, make sure you are choosing ones that are healthy, not bogged down in added sugars.

Examples of healthy snacks include:

- Hard-boiled or deviled eggs
- Almond flour crackers with almond butter
- Smoked salmon on a gluten-free cracker with dairy-free cream cheese
- Smoothies made with protein powder
- Celery sticks with a nut or seed butter
- Greek or coconut yogurt with berries
- Sugar-free turkey or beef jerky
- Olives

You can also get some great recipes and ideas using our snack section of the recipe guide at the end of the book!

Stage 1: Days 1-10

Stage one is probably the hardest phase because it is a new concept, and withdrawal will happen during this stage. You can't give up hope because there are great things to come. Let's look at what the withdrawal symptoms are one more time:

- ☐ Depressed mood
- ☐ Anxiety
- ☐ Cognitive issues – trouble concentrating
- ☐ Change in sleep pattern
- ☐ Cravings
- ☐ Light-headedness or dizziness
- ☐ Fatigue
- ☐ Nausea
- ☐ Headaches
- ☐ _____
- ☐ _____
- ☐ _____

Don't forget that everyone is different, so there may be some symptoms you won't experience. There may be some symptoms that you experience that isn't on this list, in which case there are lines you can add them in (this part will be important later on).

Setting Goals

Your body is going to go through a lot of changes during this time, so the goals you set should be obtainable for this stage of the detox process. Don't try to do too much at once during Stage 1. Stick with maybe two or three overall goals, but make sure these are goals you will be able to follow through with.

- – Possible goals for Stage 1:
- – Replace soda with water
- – Increase protein
- – Increase healthy fat intake
- – Choose fresh fruits or vegetables
- – Prioritize sleep
- – Keep healthy snacks available
- – Don't skip meals
- – Exercise more

You aren't limited to just these goals. You can come up with some of your own too. You will find that once you have goals in place, they will follow through the remaining stages. By the time you get to Stage 5, you will be able to maintain the lifestyle – if you decide that is what you want to do.

You will find that the foundation for Stages 2 through 5 are all found within this first stage. Still, they will have a different level of difficulty surrounding them. Kind of like when you begin strength training, you have to build up endurance. With my 40-day sugar detox plan, you are building up the endurance to live a life free from the added and refined sugar that once ruled your existence.

Choosing Positive Self-Affirmations

Part of being successful is having a positive outlook and self-esteem. When you feel miserable, it may be hard to see that silver lining, but I assure you it is there. Each day you will start with one or two positive self-affirmations.

What is an affirmation? Let me explain. Affirmations are the practice of positive thinking and self-empowerment. Your mind is complex. It is also capable of great things, whether you realize it or not.

Think about it using this scenario:

At some point during the night, the power went out, leaving your alarm clock flashing and an alarm that never went off. You end up waking up late for work and have to rush around to get ready. You get to your job an hour later than you would have because there was an accident on the freeway, so traffic was backed up.

In this scenario, you are probably in a bad mood. You feel like nothing is going right. The rest of your day is ruined because of these few events. What if you looked at it differently?

What if that alarm not going off saved your life. You could have been the one in the accident if you were on time. Also, you have a job which some people don't have the luxury of having. What if you came at this with a positive attitude instead of a negative one? The tone of your day could be completely different.

These are examples of affirmations:

- I am successful
- I am confident
- I am strong
- I am an unstoppable force of nature
- All I need can be found within me
- I don't need sugar to feel good
- I love myself

The list truly goes on. As long as it is a positive and uplifting statement, it can be an affirmation. You can use affirmations when you are meditating by making it your focal point. You can also recite them when you are feeling discouraged or down on yourself.

Affirmations are not an instant cure to the blues, especially not at first. Like with meditation and mindfulness, you have to train yourself and your mind.

Start a Journal

Journaling is a good way to get your feelings out. I'm talking about all feelings – anger, frustration, sadness, happiness, etc. It is a therapeutic process that can help you work through the emotions you might feel during this entire process.

Your journal doesn't have to be anything fancy. When I started this process, I was a private person. I didn't want the input from those around me, nor did I want their opinions. I wrote everything down. The closer I got to my 40-day goal, the more open I was about the experience. I realized that there aren't a lot of real-life experience out there on this subject. I wanted to bring my plan to the table without the added sugar.

Maybe you are more outspoken. In that case, you might want to try making a blog or a vlog of your journey. Making these types of posts can help someone else looking to try the same 40-day sugar detox method. These are both efficient types of journaling, which may be satisfying to the user and the audience.

Better Days Will Come

This is just the beginning of a journey that will change your life. You will begin thinking that I am insane for telling you to do some of the things I have explained. It's okay, I'll take one for the home team!

I just want to be the encouragement you need in your ear during this time. This is a hard time for you, it's like seeing the world through a whole new perspective. As you come through this first stage, you are like a newborn coming into the world. Only this world isn't overloaded with added sugars.

Stage 2: Days 11-20

Like I already said, Stage 1 is the foundation for your remaining stages. The only difference is how you approach situations. You will feel better by this point, able to focus more on the tasks at hand. The clarification alone will help you move through these days.

It is likely that you will still have some fatigue, but it will lessen as each day goes on. You may still have to mentally motivate yourself to do some morning exercises to get your blood pumping, but I have been there, and it is worth it.

Make Your Goals a Tad Harder

During the first stage, your goals were minimal, and for a good reason. The symptoms of withdrawal can make you tired and irritable. You don't want to do anything. Stage 1 is not where you want to have failures. It is where you should nurture positivity and the accomplishments that you make.

For Stage 2, increase your goals a little bit. You don't have to go to the extreme (you still have a few stages left to go). If you only had two goals during the first ten days, increase it to four goals during these ten days. You want to keep your same goals and add to them. The more you practice, the better you get!

Maintain Healthy Eating Habits

Now, more than ever, staying the course for your sugar-free lifestyle is essential. During this stage, any of the lingering withdrawal symptoms should fully subside, leaving you with a little more clarity about what sugar was doing to your life. The same goes for giving up carbohydrates. Your body goes through a process before becoming better.

It is easy to fall back into old habits when you aren't feeling the withdrawal symptoms anymore. You will feel like you are on top of the world, but if you caved now, your body would likely experience some repercussions from the sugar shock.

Keep Up with Your Journal, Blog, Vlog, Whatever!

Your experience is likely different from my experience. Your experience is likely different from Joe Shmo from Kokomo's. I wrote a book about my 40-day sugar detox to help guide you. You can use your journal (if you want) to guide others based on your experiences.

There is not enough information readily available to the masses to help them make the decisions they need to make about this lifestyle change. You can be a voice to that, just like me! If you can laugh about it and present it in a positive light, your audience will thank you.

Increase Your Physical Activity

Your body is resetting itself now that the sugar is leaving it. This is your chance to swoop in and increase your endorphins by increasing your physical activity. Doing this will let you experience your body's natural energy system and "feel good" hormones. You will see that the sugar high is nothing compared to what endorphins create.

As you increase your physical activity, you need to increase your protein and healthy fats. These will help with your metabolism and energy but burn at a slower rate than the sugar did. You will feel energized longer. The protein will also help your muscles recover after a workout.

Stage 3: Days 21-30

Get ready for the longest ten days of your life. I'm not saying this to be discouraging, but you are going to need to get creative if you want to stay motivated. Your goals need to be more challenging at this point. You have already made it through the withdrawals, but you are likely still experiencing some cravings. They may be more noticeable when you go out with people who aren't sharing the same philosophy that you have right now.

I wish I could say that this will go away, but all I can offer is that it does get better. You will also become creative, finding things on the menu that you had never noticed before. To help yourself out, most restaurants have a low-carb section. It is within this section that you will find your top meal contenders. Sugars are carbs, so fewer carbs mean less sugar. You may even find that some places have a sugar-free menu that you can ask for, this doesn't always happen, but the worst they can tell you is that they don't have one!

Decide on a Big Goal for Day 40

I didn't bring this up before now because you have to crawl before you can walk, and you have to walk before you can run. Now that you are halfway through the detox, you can set your sights on something a little bigger.

Before setting your Stage 3 goals in stone, come up with the big goal for the end. You may need to use your goals for this set of days to prepare for your overall goal. For example, if you want to run a 5K, you will want to start conditioning as soon as possible – these can be your goals for this stage.

Obviously, it is unlikely that there will be a 5K scheduled on your day 40, wherever it may fall, but you can set your small goals to help you meet the big one. I'm not saying you have to do a 5K as your big goal. It's only an example. Do something that you love to do.

Create Your Stage 3 Goals

You have come quite a way from day 1, and you need to look at that with an appreciation for yourself. All of the goals you make should be for you, not for anyone else. Increase your goals during these ten days. You are at a point where you probably feel like you have done this forever, and you are cured. You aren't cured, though, so don't think about calling it a day.

Keep the momentum going by increasing your workout routine. Switch it up and try something you have never done before. Take a dance class. Go to a yoga class. Take a beginner's class because no one knows what they are doing. I found that I was great at the "rolling log." Yeah, no one at the class found that joke funny, either.

The bottom line, open yourself up to new experiences and stop playing it safe. Safe was stuffing your face with snack cakes watching primetime television. Now, you are taking the world by storm, telling sugar where to stick it. You don't need those snack cakes anymore!

Talk About Your Experiences

You should be in a good place at this point in the process to open up and talk about it if you want to. No one will force you to share your sugar detox experiences if you don't want to. Other people may have questions, and since you are going through the process, you might be the best spokesperson.

I'm mainly referring to online forums and such. The last time I checked, there wasn't a local sugar addicts anonymous chapter support group. Online forums are just as beneficial, though. Think about where you were two weeks ago, imagine how someone who doesn't have a support group might feel. This opportunity could allow you to connect with others choosing a sugar-free lifestyle.

Stage 4: Days 31-40

The finish line is in sight. Your last ten days of the actual sugar detox plan are among you. By day 40, you will have a decision to make, but since we aren't there, we won't dwell too much on it quite yet. I commend you for your strength and courage to kick sugar to the curb. You have done so well, and you deserve all the rewards you have waiting for you at the end!

You are preparing for your big goal at the end of this program, which is exciting for you. You still need to set some other goals, which can be related to your overall goal, and follow through to the finish. These days will fly by, and you will be at the end before you know it. Sure, the last ten days seemed to take forever. These will feel like they never happened at all!

Don't Quit Because You Feel Ahead

Now is not the time to get cocky. Just because you are ahead in the final quarter doesn't mean you can't lose the game. How many times have you watched a sporting event and your team was ahead only to lose during the final seconds of the game?

You have come a long way, but unless you finish, you can't feel accomplished. Sure, you could stop now and go on with your life, remaining sugar-free, but unless you close the chapter on sugar, it will remain a lingering thought you can't shake.

Plan on finishing strong these last ten days. I believe in you, so you should believe in you too!

Start Thinking About the Future

You still have a few days before you reach the finish line. You have learned a lot throughout this journey. The lessons you learned are something that can stick with you for the rest of your life if you will let them.

- By this point, you are feeling accomplished in all the things you have done so far. Accomplishment brings about a sense of pride, which you have every right to feel. When I was doing this same program, I found that pride was what kept me going—knowing that I had accomplished what I set out to do made it worth it.
- Hopefully, your self-esteem is higher now than it was when you started on day 1. You aren't being pulled down by the weight of the simple carbohydrates anymore, and you can feel more like yourself.
- Plus side, you have probably lost weight without planning on it. That helps with your self-esteem too, but even more, it makes you healthier.

Where do you want to go from here? Do you want to keep with this type of lifestyle? Do you want to backslide a little, have the occasional sugary treat every now and then?

I thought I was in the latter scenario. I thought just a little bit every now and then won't hurt anything. I have come so far. Nothing will set me back. I'm going to give you a cold, honest truth right now. As a sugar addict, there is never an "occasional sugary treat."

I'm not saying this to kick you in the gut when you are close to the finish line. I'm sharing the truth about being an addict. Once in a while turns into sometimes, which turns into every other day, then it's your daily reward. You could potentially ruin the progress you made in less time than it took to get where you are.

Constantly Acknowledge the Home Stretch

The home stretch during stage 4 is an accomplishment. Consider the last week of your detox the final lap, you have completed all the required laps for the checkered flag to be brought out. No more caution flags, no more pit stops, this is it – you are doing this.

You have to take this time to be proud of yourself. Talk about the accomplishments you have made. Share how much better you feel with those around you. You may not have had the most encouraging support over these last 40 days, especially those who don't understand why you chose to change your lifestyle.

They don't have to understand as long as you understand. You can share with them at this point how your mental clarity has become more open and you understand that you were addicted, poisoning yourself with sugar. Sugar controlled you worse than any other habit you have.

Explaining these changes, you feel should be easier now, because people are going to begin seeing them, they are also going to be evident to you. Your skin will feel smoother, your confidence higher, and possibly a smaller waistline to boot. You changed and you had the power to do it without being forced to do it.

Use the accomplishments you have made to be your swan song to the first 40 days of detox. You have a big decision coming up, but you shouldn't have to worry about it just yet. You have to decide if you are going to keep the lifestyle change or revert back to the sugary ways of the world – maybe even a hybrid version, whatever that may be.

I do implore you, think long and hard before you make too drastic of a decision that could require you to have to repeat this process all over again. Weigh out the pros and cons, and maybe it can be just one of those things where you do it on special occasions. Even I understand that it is hard to celebrate with people and not be able to eat the cake, just don't eat the whole cake in a blind sugar rage!

Stage 5: Days 41+Beyond

CONGRATULATIONS!!! You have made it to Stage 5 – from here, it is up to you where you go. You single-handedly took the step 40 days ago to change your life. Do you feel different? Take a moment to look back over the stages you successfully made it through. Do you remember how it felt on that first day versus where you are right now?

Do a simple self-evaluation:

Question	Answer
Do I feel better than I felt on the day I began the 40-day sugar detox plan?	
What were the challenges that I faced? How did I overcome them?	
The worst part about this experience was...	
The best part about this experience was...	
Did you meet each of the goals you made for yourself?	

What advice do you have for someone who wants to do this plan?

The answers to the evaluation should help you decide if you want to go forward with your sugar-free lifestyle. My goal is to help you continue this lifestyle so that you can feel better and healthier on a daily basis.

I don't know if you know it, but many of the things you love are also available in a sugar-free form – you just need to keep an eye on the amount of artificial sweetener you eat. These could be just what you need to satisfy a lingering sweet tooth or even for a big shindig!

How to Create a Plan Going Forward

Your plan going forward will be like the ones you did for the 40-day plan, but less invasive. You won't need to list your goals unless you find yourself beginning to slack. Keep up with your journal, and keep up with the food planning parts of the program. These are what will help you remain accountable and keep your meals sugar-free and healthy.

- Make your shopping list based on your meal plan. Don't purchase things that aren't on the list unless they fit in with the sugar-free lifestyle.
- Don't give up if you fall off the wagon. At this point, you should have an easier time getting back on it.

- Find yourself a way to cope when things get stressful – go for a jog, take a walk, listen to music, etc. Always have an emergency plan!
- Constantly look for ways to make your changes worth it. Share your story, create a blog, or you could write your story!

It isn't about how far you have come. It's about where you are going. You made it through a jungle of sugar addiction, and now you are living cleaner and healthier. Make sure you celebrate your accomplishments.

My 40-Day Detox

It is one thing for me to tell you how to handle a 40-day detox, but it means nothing if I don't tell you my story. Why should you listen to some random lady who is telling you that the sugar is the devil? I get it which is why I'm going to give you some insight on my journey.

Before I began my 40 days, there was a lot of denial. **I wasn't an addict**. That was what I told myself at least. There was no way that I was an addict – I didn't smoke, do drugs, or drink alcohol. There was no reason to place me in that category, I simply ate too much sugar and my health was at risk.

I didn't admit the truth until I was well into the withdrawal process. I knew that if it was that difficult for me, I had a problem that I wasn't admitting. Needless to say, there were some setbacks during that time, but I finally got through it.

I had to change how I thought about the entire process. Even though I used online resources and articles, I didn't have "me" to guide myself through the process. I was flying blind into a world that was unfamiliar.

That was when I started keeping a journal. I wanted to be able to share how I was feeling and make notes that might help others get through the emotions they were feeling if they were in my position. I didn't want to forget how I felt during the process, because if I ever chose to go back to my old lifestyle, I could read it and remember exactly what I went through to get where I was.

I won't pretend that the journey was easy because it wasn't. But I can say with some certainty, 40 days can change your life.

Do It For Yourself

People come up with all kinds of reasons about why they start a diet or make a lifestyle change. These changes usually revolve around pleasing someone else. I'm here to tell you that the only way you are going to be successful is if you do this for yourself.

Do this for your health – so that you are here for your children, husband, etc.

Do this for your mental health – so that you are more calm and easier to be around.

Do this because you want to accomplish it – and show those around you that you can do anything you put your mind to.

Don't do this because someone isn't attracted to you. Don't do this because someone told you that you could be at risk of health problems, but you lack the motivation. Don't let anyone be your motivation, except for you.

Harsh? Probably. The truth? Absolutely. I spent years, especially in high school, trying to please others. I wanted to be the one that people liked. I wanted to be the one with the popular boyfriend. I wanted to wear a size 0 and hang out at the mall.

I was smart and I was liked, for my brains, not my looks. I wasn't a size 0, sure there is a 0 in my size, it just doesn't fly solo. I didn't have the popular boyfriend, instead I surrounded myself with like-minded chess nerds.

Do I regret any of it? Yes. I regret that I felt like I had to be someone that I wasn't for other people. I regret that I didn't think more of myself. It didn't stop there through.

Be honest with me, how much do you think of yourself? I mean how nice are you to yourself? Probably not very good, right? When you make these changes, you will begin to feel more accomplished and really good about yourself.

So, my biggest piece of advice is to do it for yourself – and leave others to their own problems.

DAY	HOW DO I FEEL?	MY POSITIVE AFFIRMATIONS	NOTES

My Goals:

Chapter Seven: Recipes, Snacks, and Making It

You have to eat, even if you are steering clear of the sugar. Collecting different recipes for your breakfast, lunch, dinner, side dishes, and snacks can help you prepare your meals in advance so you aren't trying to make last-minute dinner decisions. When you are in a rush, you can end up turning to foods that are high in added sugar because they are easier.

I'm going to help you become an expert at planning your low and sugar-free menu and plans. Being organized is one way that I found to help with my transition. Here is how you can make your plan (if you want it to be done weekly):

	Meal	**Shopping List**
Sunday		
Monday		
Tuesday		
Wednesday		
Thursday		
Friday		
Saturday		

Using a plan like this can help you with planning your shopping list, too. You can look at the recipes or list the items you need to make a special dish in the last column, which will let you know what you need to purchase.

To make identifying special characteristics of the recipe easier, I have included a key to illustrate these features.

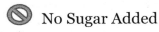 No Sugar Added

Sugar-Free

Gluten-Free

Dairy-Free

Vegetarian

Vegan

Breakfast Recipes

Breakfast is the most important meal of the day – at least that is what they say! I have picked out some of the recipes that will make your morning easier and are delicious while keeping you on track with your sugar detox.

Cottage Cheese Pancakes

Prep Time: 3 minutes
Cook Time: 9 minutes
Yield: 1 pancake

Ingredients:
1 tsp olive oil or butter
½ cup cottage cheese
3 eggs
½ cup rolled oats

Instructions:
1. For this step you can use a bowl or a blender. Mix together all of the ingredients until smooth.
2. Heat a pan with a small amount of oil on low to medium heat, add the batter.
3. Flip once bubble start to appear. Cook until both sides are golden brown.

Nutrition:

Serving Size	1 pancake		
Calories	481	Potassium	438mg
Fat	24g	Carbohydrates	32g
Saturated Fat	9g	Fiber	4g
Cholesterol	520mg	Sugar	4g
Sodium	608mg	Protein	34g

PB Cup Smoothie

Prep Time: N/A
Cook Time: Less than 5 minutes
Yield: 1 Smoothie

Ingredients:
1 tsp vanilla extract
1 Tbsp unsweetened cocoa powder
1 large ripe banana, peeled, cut into chunks, frozen
1 ½ Tbsp natural peanut butter
½ cup plain 2% Greek Yogurt
1 cup unsweetened almond milk

Directions:
1. Add all ingredients to a blender, puree until smooth
2. Serve or refrigerate until ready to serve

Nutrition:

Serving Size	1 smoothie
Calories	408
Fat	18g
Saturated Fat	4g
Carbohydrates	43g
Sugar	21g
Fiber	8g
Protein	19g

Paleo Minute English Muffins

Prep Time: 1 minute
Cook Time: 1 minute
Yield: 1 muffin – 2 servings

Ingredients:
1/8 tsp salt
1 Tbsp coconut flour
¼ tsp baking powder
1 egg
1 ½ tsp coconut oil
1 ½ Tbsp almond butter

Directions:
1. Stir the coconut oil, egg, and almond butter together until well combined in a mug.
2. Stir in the coconut flour, salt, and baking powder.
3. Microwave on HIGH for 1 to 1 ½ minutes.
4. Remove from the mug and slice in half.

Nutrition:

Serving Size	1 slice		
Calories	146	Potassium	170mg
Fat	12g	Carbohydrates	4g
Saturated Fat	4g	Fiber	2g
Cholesterol	81mg	Sugar	0g
Sodium	185mg	Protein	5g

No Egg Breakfast Bake

Could be dairy-free if no cheese used

Prep Time: 10 minutes
Cook Time: 40 minutes
Yield: 4 servings

Ingredients:

½ cup grated mozzarella cheese (optional if dairy-free)
1 large green bell pepper, cleaned and chopped
1 large red bell pepper, cleaned and chopped
10 oz. pre-cooked turkey or pork breakfast sausage links
1 ½ tsp olive oil
All-purpose seasoning of choice to taste
Ground black pepper to taste

Directions:

1. Preheat your oven to 450°F
2. Spray a medium sized baking or casserole dish with non-stick spray.
3. Add the chopped peppers to the baking dish with 1 tsp olive oil and sprinkle with spices. Place the dish in the oven and bake for 20 minutes.
4. While cooking peppers, place the remaining ½ tsp of olive oil in a pan and cook the sausage over medium-high heat approximately 10 to 12 minutes or until browned.
5. Cut the sausage into thirds.
6. Remove the peppers from the oven and add the sausages to the dish. Bake an additional five minutes.
7. OPTIONAL – Remove the dish from the oven and turn to broil. Sprinkle the grated mozzarella cheese over the peppers and sausage. Return to the oven and broil for an additional one to two minutes, or until the cheese is melted.

Nutrition:

Serving Size	¼ piece		
Calories	246	Carbohydrates	5g
Fat	13g	Fiber	1g
Saturated Fat	5g	Sugar	2g
Cholesterol	98mg	Protein	26g
Sodium	351mg		

Cheesy Egg Muffins with Green Chiles

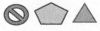

Prep Time: 5 minutes
Cook Time: 35 minutes
Yield: 12 medium-sized muffins

Ingredients:
¾ cup sliced green onions
2 tsp Spike spice or equivalent
2 cans (4oz each) diced green chiles, drained
15 eggs
3 cups Mexican Blend Cheese
Salt and pepper to taste

Directions:
1. Preheat oven to 375°F
2. Spray baking tins or cups with non-stick cooking spray
3. In each cup put some cheese, diced green chiles, and onion
4. Beat the eggs until well combined. Add the spices to the eggs.
5. Pour the eggs into each cup until full
6. Using a fork, gently stir each cup to mix contents
7. Bake for 35 minutes or until all muffins have puffed up and appear to be golden. These will last for up to a week in the refrigerator.

Nutrition:

Serving Size	1 muffin		
Calories	194	Carbohydrates	2g
Fat	14g	Fiber	0g
Saturated Fat	7g	Sugar	1g
Cholesterol	259mg	Protein	15g
Sodium	486mg		

Shamrock Breakfast Sandwich

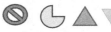

Prep Time: 5 minutes
Cook Time: 10 minutes
Yield: 1 serving

Ingredients:
2 tsp extra virgin olive oil
1 vegan sausage patty
1 Tbsp pepitas
1 cup kale
Salt and pepper to taste
1 English muffin, toasted
¼ avocado, sliced
Sauce:
$1/8$ tsp chipotle powder or smoky paprika
1 Tbsp vegan mayo
1 tsp jalapeno, chopped – optional

Directions:
1. Add a little of the oil to a sauté pan and preheat on high heat. Cook the vegan sausage patty one to two minutes and flip.
2. Add the kale and pepitas to the pan, toasting the pepitas and wilting the kale. Add salt and pepper to taste. When vegan sausage patty is browned and the kale is soft, turn off heat.
3. Mix together the ingredients for the sauce.
4. Assemble all of the items on top of the English muffin. Serve warm for best results.

Nutrition:

Serving Size	1 sandwich		
Calories	573	Carbohydrates	44g
Fat	35g	Fiber	8g
Saturated Fat	5g	Sugar	1g
Protein	21g	Potassium	823mg
Sodium	707mg		

Simple Breakfast Hash

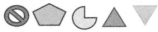

Prep Time: 15 minutes
Cook Time: 45 minutes
Yield: 6 servings

Ingredients:
3 medium russet potatoes, peeled and diced
1 large, sweet potato, peeled and diced
¼ cup olive oil + 1 tsp olive oil
2 tsp sea salt
1 tsp pepper
1 Tbsp onion powder
1 Tbsp garlic powder
1 tsp dried thyme
1 medium onion, diced
5 cloves garlic, finely diced or minced

Directions:
1. Preheat oven to 450°F spray a cooking dish with non-stick cooking spray
2. Combine the diced potatoes, ¼ cup olive oil, and spices. Mix well and add to the cooking dish. Bake for 40 to 50 minutes, stirring every 20 minutes or until crispy.
3. Sauté onion, 1 tsp olive oil, and garlic in a skillet. Cook for 5 to 8 minutes or until browned.
4. Once potatoes are crispy, remove from the oven and stir in the skillet mixture until combined.
5. Serve warm.

Nutrition:

Serving Size	¹/₆ portion		
Calories	212	Carbohydrates	28g
Fat	10g	Fiber	4g
Saturated Fat	1g	Sugar	3g
Protein	3g	Cholesterol	0mg
Sodium	781mg		

Egg White Frittata

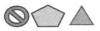

Prep Time: 10 minutes
Cook Time: 10 minutes
Yield: 2 large servings

Ingredients:
1 red pepper, cleaned and chopped
¼ yellow onion, chopped
1 green pepper, cleaned and chopped
2 Tbsp olive oil
1 tsp kosher salt
1 tsp black pepper
8 egg whites
2 cups fresh spinach
½ cup feta cheese, crumbled

Directions:
1. Preheat oven to 375°F
2. In a skillet, add the olive oil and preheat over medium-low heat. Add the onions and peppers, sauté approximately 7 minutes until tender. Sprinkle with salt and pepper.
3. Pour the egg whites into the skillet and cook for three minutes. Sprinkle the feta and spinach on the mixture.
4. Put the skillet into the oven and bake uncovered for 8 to 10 minutes. Loosen with spatula and invert onto a serving plate.

Nutrition:

Serving Size	½ frittata		
Calories	300	Potassium	646mg
Fat	20.8g	Carbohydrates	11.2g
Saturated Fat	5.6g	Fiber	4.2g
Cholesterol	20mg	Sugar	5.5g
Sodium	1160mg	Protein	21.6g

Black Forest Turkey with Egg Cups

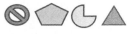

Prep Time: N/A
Cook Time: 25 minutes + 5-10 cooling
Yield: 10-12

Ingredients:
2 green onions, chopped
2 medium zucchinis, shredded
¼ cup chopped parsley
3 cloves of garlic, minced
10 eggs
$^1/_8$ tsp celery or regular salt
4 to 6 oz black forest turkey, uncured, natural

Directions:
1. Preheat oven to 350°F. Grease a muffin tin.
2. Whisk the 10 eggs together in a large bowl
3. Add the vegetables and seasonings to the eggs, stir to combine.
4. Line each of the muffin cups with a piece of the turkey and fill with ¼ cup of the egg mixture.
5. Bake for 25 minutes. Cool before serving.

Nutrition:

Serving Size	1 egg cup		
Calories	76	Potassium	149mg
Fat	3.8g	Carbohydrates	2.1g
Saturated Fat	1.2g	Fiber	.5g
Cholesterol	141mg	Sugar	.9g
Sodium	124mg	Protein	8.3g

Clean Eating Black Bean Scramble

Prep Time: 10 minutes
Cook Time: 15 minutes
Yield: 1 serving

Ingredients:
½ cup black beans, no sugar added
4 large eggs
$^1/_3$ medium avocado
¼ medium onion, chopped
½ tsp olive oil
2 Tbsp salsa, no sugar added

Directions:
1. Sauté onions in the oil using a non-stick frying pan
2. Add the eggs to the skillet and cook/scramble
3. When eggs are close to done, add the beans and cook to heat up
4. Transfer to a plate, serve topped with avocado and salsa

Nutrition:

Serving Size	1 scramble		
Calories	212	Potassium	604mg
Fat	3g	Carbohydrates	23g
Sodium	428mg	Fiber	8g
Sugar	2g		
Protein	22g		

Lunch Recipes

It will become apparent how important it is to eat three meals a day during your detox. Here are some lunch recipes that you can use to limit the amount of sugar you intake. These are good for at home or on the go!

Greek Orzo Salad

Prep Time: 10 minutes
Cook Time: 10 minutes
Yield: 6 servings

Ingredients:
$1/3$ cup olive oil
1 clove garlic, minced
3 Tbsp fresh lemon juice
Salt and pepper to taste
1 cup feta cheese
1 ¼ cup dry orzo
1 medium English cucumber, diced
1 (10.5 oz) pkg. grape tomatoes, halved
½ cup chopped red onion, rinsed
½ cup kalamata olives, sliced
2 Tbsp fresh parsley, chopped
3 Tbsp fresh basil, chopped

Directions:
1. In a jar, mix the olive oil, lemon juice, garlic, salt, and pepper. Set the mixture to the side.
2. Cook the orzo according to the directions on the package. Drain and allow to cool about five minutes.
3. Add all of the ingredients together in a large bowl, including the orzo. Add the mixture from the jar and toss to evenly coat. Keep refrigerated.

Nutrition:

Serving Size	1 serving		
Calories	320	Potassium	199mg
Fat	19g	Carbohydrates	28g
Saturated Fat	5g	Fiber	1g
Cholesterol	22mg	Sugar	3g
Sodium	458mg	Protein	8g

Grilled Buffalo Chicken in Lettuce Wraps

Prep Time: 35 minutes
Cook Time: 10 minutes
Cook Time: 10 minutes
Yield: 15-20 wraps

Ingredients:
3 large boneless, skinless chicken breasts, cut into ½"
cubes
15-20 butter lettuce cups
¾ cup Frank's Red Hot Sauce
1 avocado, diced
¾ cup cherry tomatoes, halved
½ cup ranch dressing
¼ cup sliced green onions

Instructions:
1. Place ½ cup of the Frank's Red Hot Sauce in a bowl with
the chicken. Cover and place in the refrigerator to marinate
for 30 minutes.
2. Preheat grill to 400°F
3. Using a grill basket or kabob sticks, grill the marinated
chicken for 8 to 10 minutes.
4. Remove the chicken from the grill and toss in a bowl with
the remaining ¼ cup of sauce.
5. In each lettuce wrap, place 2-3 cubes of chicken, 2-3
tomatoes, 2-3 avocados, a pinch of the green onions, and
drizzle with ranch dressing.

Nutrition:

Serving Size	1 lettuce wrap		
Calories	53	Carbohydrates	2g
Fat	3g	Fiber	1g
Cholesterol	11mg	Sugar	3g
Sodium	412mg	Protein	5g

BLT Chicken Salad

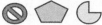

Total Time: 20 minutes
Yield: 8 servings

Ingredients:
½ cup mayonnaise
2 Tbsp onion, finely chopped
3-4 Tbsp barbeque sauce
1 Tbsp lemon juice
¼ tsp pepper
2 large tomatoes, chopped
8 cups torn salad greens
10 strips bacon, cooked and crumbled
1 ½ pounds chicken breast, boneless, skinless, cooked and cubed
2 hard-boiled eggs, sliced

Directions:
1. In a small bowl, combine the mayonnaise, onion, barbeque sauce, lemon juice, and pepper. Cover and refrigerate until ready to serve salad.
2. In a large bowl, fill with the salad greens. Sprinkle the tomatoes, chicken, and bacon on top of the greens. Garnish with the sliced eggs. Drizzle the dressing you made and toss to coat.

Nutrition:

Serving Size	1 serving		
Calories	281	Carbohydrates	5g
Fat	19g	Fiber	2g
Saturated Fat	4g	Sugar	3g
Cholesterol	112mg	Protein	23g

Garden Frittata

Prep Time: 25 minutes
Cook Time: 45 minutes + standing
Yield: 6 servings

Ingredients:
1 small zucchini, thinly sliced
1 small yellow summer squash, thinly sliced
1 cup shredded part-skim mozzarella cheese
1 small onion, chopped
¼ cup crumbled feta cheese
1 medium tomato, sliced
4 large eggs
2 Tbsp fresh basil, minced
1 cup fat-free milk
½ tsp salt
1 clove garlic, minced
¼ tsp pepper
¼ cup shredded parmesan cheese

Directions:

1. Preheat oven to 375°F and coat a 9" pie plate with non-stick cooking spray
2. In a microwave safe bowl, mix the squash, zucchini, and onion. Cover and microwave on high for 7 to 9 minutes or until the vegetables are tender. Drain excess water.
3. Place the vegetables in the pie plate. Top with mozzarella, feta, and tomato.
4. In a large bowl, whisk the eggs, basil, milk, garlic, salt, and pepper. Pour this mixture over the cheese and tomato layer. Sprinkle the parmesan cheese on top.
5. Bake uncovered for 45 to 50 minutes, or until a knife inserted into the center comes out clean. Let it stand at least 10 minutes before cutting into 6 pieces and serving.

Nutrition:

Serving Size	1 serving		
Calories	161	Carbohydrates	7g
Fat	9g	Fiber	1g
Saturated Fat	4g	Sugar	5g
Cholesterol	142mg	Protein	13g
Sodium	494mg		

Cauliflower Pizza Lunch Muffins

Prep Time: 20 minutes
Cook Time: 25 minutes
Yield: 12 muffins

Ingredients:
3 large eggs
3 cups riced cauliflower
½ tsp salt
1 tsp dried oregano
1 tsp dried basil
¾ cup almond flour
1 ½ cups shredded cheese + ½ cup shredded cheese
½ tsp baking powder
12 tsp pizza sauce

Directions:
1. Preheat oven to 350°F. Line a muffin pan with parchment paper or spray with non-stick cooking spray.
2. In a large bowl, combine the cauliflower, salt, basil, eggs, 1 ½ cups shredded cheese, eggs, oregano, almond flour, and baking powder.
3. Divide between 12 muffin cups. Top each of the muffin mixture with 1 tsp pizza sauce and sprinkle with remaining cheese.
4. Bake in oven for 25 to 28 minutes, until thoroughly cooked.

Nutrition:

Serving Size	1 muffin		
Calories	164	Potassium	205mg
Fat	12g	Carbohydrates	4g
Saturated Fat	4g	Fiber	1g
Cholesterol	64mg	Sugar	1g
Sodium	414mg	Protein	9g

Turkey Pesto Cucumber Roll-ups

Prep Time: 15 minutes
Cook Time: N/A
Yield: 18 roll-ups

Ingredients:
¼ cup store-bought basil pesto
3 medium cucumbers
6 Vegan Mozzarella Slices, cut into ½" strips
1 bell pepper, thinly sliced
6 oz deli-smoked turkey
½ cup spinach, shredded
Salt and pepper to taste

Directions:
1. Slice the cucumber lengthwise using a mandoline on 2mm setting. If you do not have one, you can use a vegetable peeler. Place the slices on parchment paper and pat dry.
2. Spread about 1 tsp of pesto on each slice of cucumber. Spread it and place cheese, turkey, bell pepper, and spinach evenly on each slice. Sprinkle each with salt and pepper.
3. Roll each slice with the contents, creating a roll-up. Use a toothpick to keep together for a cleaner appearance.

Nutrition:

Serving Size	1 roll-up		
Calories	52	Carbohydrates	2.5g
Fat	3g	Sugar	1.1g
Protein	3.8g		

Cold Lemon Zoodles

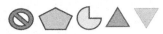

Prep Time: 20 minutes
Cook Time: N/A
Yield: 4 servings

Ingredients:
½ tsp Dijon mustard
1 lemon, zested and juiced
$^1/_3$ cup olive oil
½ tsp garlic powder
3 medium zucchinis, cut into noodles
1 Tbsp fresh thyme, chopped
1 bunch radishes, thinly sliced
Salt and pepper to taste

Directions:
1. In a small bowl, combine the lemon zest, mustard, lemon juice, and garlic powder, whisk together.
2. Add in the olive oil and continue to whisk. Season with the salt and pepper.
3. In a large bowl, toss together the zucchini noodles with the radishes. Add the dressing you just made and toss with the vegetables in the bowl.
4. Use fresh thyme to garnish.

Nutrition:

Serving Size	1 serving		
Calories	198	Carbohydrates	8g
Fat	19g	Sugar	5g
Protein	2g		

Nori Vegetable Rolls

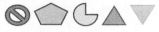

Yield: 1 roll

Ingredients:
2 Tbsp hummus
1 sheet nori
¼ cup shredded carrots
¼ cup sweet pea shoots or sprouts
1 Tbsp nutritional yeast flakes
¼ avocado, thinly sliced
1 small Persian cucumber, sliced to matchstick size
1 tsp lemon juice
Salt to taste

Directions:
1. Arrange your nori sheet on a flat working area with the long edge close to you.
2. Spread out the hummus in a thin layer over the nori sheet.
3. Layer the carrots, pea shoots, cucumber, and avocado on top the bottom third of the nori. Sprinkle with the lemon juice and salt to taste.
4. Gently and firmly begin rolling the nori sheet. You can use a bamboo sushi mat for assistance.
5. Cut the roll in to smaller pieces using a sharp knife. Serve immediately or refrigerate.

Nutrition:

Serving Size	1 serving		
Calories	276	Carbohydrates	15.8g
Fat	18.4g	Sugar	4.1g
Protein	17.5g	Sodium	488.6mg

Spinach Stuffed Cremini Mushrooms with Feta

Prep Time: 10 minutes
Cook Time: 20 minutes
Yield: 6 servings

Ingredients:
8 oz spinach, chopped
1 Tbsp olive oil
1 pound Cremini mushrooms, stems removed
½ cup feta cheese, crumbled
1 Tbsp fresh parsley, minced
4 cloves garlic, minced
Salt and pepper to taste

Directions:
1. Preheat oven to 400°F. Line a baking sheet with aluminum foil or parchment paper. If using aluminum foil, grease surface lightly.
2. In a bowl, place the spinach and a few Tbsp of water, cover with plastic wrap. Steam in the microwave for two minutes, until wilted. Drain excess water.
3. Arrange the mushrooms with the bottom facing up on the pan. Drizzle with the olive oil and sprinkle with salt and pepper.
4. When spinach has cooled, squeeze by hand to release extra water.
5. Mix the feta, spinach, garlic, and parsley in a bowl. Spoon into the mushroom's cavities.
6. Bake for 15 to 20 minutes, until the mushrooms are soft and golden brown.

Nutrition:

Serving Size	4 mushrooms		
Calories	82.2	Carbohydrates	5.5g
Fat	5.4g	Sugar	2.6g
Protein	4.6g	Fiber	1.9g

Avocado Egg Salad

Prep Time: 10 minutes
Yield: 6 servings

Ingredients:
3 Tbsp lime juice
2 medium avocados
¾ tsp sea salt
3 Tbsp red onion, minced
¼ cup cilantro
1 Tbsp jalapenos, minced
3 Tbsp celery, finely chopped
8 large hard boiled eggs, diced

Directions:
1. Mash the avocado and lime juice together. Add in the salt and leave some chunks of avocado present.
2. Fold in the red onion, cilantro, celery, and jalapenos. Stir until combined.
3. Gently fold in the eggs, mashing yolks as you go. Add additional salt or jalapeno to taste. Serve plain or with favorite no-sugar added, gluten-free bread option.

Nutrition:

Serving Size	1 serving		
Calories	216	Carbohydrates	7.9g
Fat	16.9g	Sugar	1.7g
Protein	9.9g	Fiber	4.7g

Dinner Recipes

Whether it is dinner for two or dinner for the whole family, you can create masterpieces that everyone can enjoy. There are many different types of dinner dishes that can be made to keep the sugar cravings away and still taste great!

Rosemary Garlic Pork Tenderloin

Prep Time: 5 minutes
Cook Time: 16 minutes
Yield: 4 servings

Ingredients:
1 pound pork tenderloin, boneless, trimmed
¼ tsp black pepper
1 tsp salt
4 cloves garlic, crushed
3 Tbsp olive oil (divided 2 Tbsp and 1 Tbsp)
1 tsp Italian seasoning
1 Tbsp fresh rosemary, chopped
½ tsp lemon zest

Directions:
1. Preheat oven to 400°F
2. Season the pork with the salt and pepper on both sides
3. In a small bowl, stir together 2 Tbsp olive oil, fresh rosemary, garlic, lemon zest, and Italian seasoning. Brush the mixture over the pork on all sides.
4. Heat the remaining olive oil in a cast iron skillet over medium-high heat. Add the tenderloin and sear for 3 to 4 minutes without moving until it is browned on the bottom. Flip and sear the other side.
5. Place the skillet in the oven and roast for 10 to 15 minutes, or until the internal temperature of the pork reaches 145°F
6. Remove the tenderloin from the oven and let it rest for five minutes.

Nutritional:

Serving Size	¼ pound		
Calories	236	Carbohydrates	2g
Fat	15g	Fiber	1g
Protein	24g	Sugar	1g

Lamb Kofta Kebab

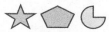

Prep Time: 10 minutes
Cook Time: 6 minutes
Yield: 8 servings

Ingredients:
8 bamboo skewers
2 cloves garlic, minced
¼ cup onion, grated
1 Tbsp fresh parsley, chopped
1 tsp cumin
1 Tbsp fresh dill, chopped
1 ½ tsp salt
¼ tsp black pepper
2 pounds ground lamb

Directions:
1. Soak the bamboo skewers in water for 30 minutes, pat dry.
2. In a large bowl, stir together all the ingredients except for the lamb. Add the lamb and mix until just combined, do not over mix this
3. Divide the meat into 16 sections. Mold each section of the meat around the skewer. Make it a few inches long and about 1 inch thick. You should put two pieces of meat per skewer.
4. Preheat the grill to medium-high heat and oil grates lightly. Place the skewers on the grill and cook for 3 minutes. Flip and cook for an additional 3 to 5 minutes, to the desired level of doneness.

Nutritional:

Serving Size	1 skewer		
Calories	324	Carbohydrates	0g
Fat	26g	Fiber	0g
Protein	18g	Sugar	0g

Mexican Skillet Zucchini

Prep Time: 5 minutes
Cook Time: 10 minutes
Yield: 4 servings

Ingredients:
1 Tbsp extra virgin olive oil
1 garlic clove, finely chopped
1 pound zucchini, diced
1 green onion, thinly sliced
1 large tomato, cored, seeded, diced
1 tsp pickled jalapeno, minced
1 Tbsp fresh cilantro minced
½ cup queso blanco or queso fresco, crumbled
Fresh lime juice, salt, and pepper, to taste

Directions:
1. In a large skillet over medium heat, cook the garlic in oil for 1 minute, stirring until it sizzles.
2. Add zucchini and cook, stirring occasionally. Continue to cook about 3 minutes or until slightly softened.
3. Add the green onion and tomatoes, cook an additional 3 minutes.
4. Remove the skillet from the heat, adding the cilantro, lime juice, and jalapeno.
5. Season with the salt and pepper to taste, topping with queso.

Nutritional:

Serving Size	¼ mixture		
Calories	102	Carbohydrates	8g
Fat	6g	Fiber	2g
Protein	5g	Sugar	3g
Cholesterol	17mg	Sodium	211mg

Grilled Garlic and Herb Chicken with Vegetables

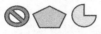

Total Time: 20 minutes
Yield: 6 servings

Ingredients:
1 ½ pounds thinly sliced chicken cutlets, boneless and skinless
Kosher salt
3 oz package garlic and herb veggie marinade
1 medium zucchini, sliced ¼" thick
1 pounds asparagus, tough ends removed
1 red bell pepper, seeded and sliced into strips
1 medium yellow squash, sliced ¼" thick
Olive oil cooking spray

Directions:
1. Season the chicken with ½ tsp salt and 2 Tbsp veggie herb marinade for at least one hour or up to all night.
2. Use the remaining marinade to marinate the veggies.
3. Heat a grill over medium-heat. Oil grates to prevent sticking.
4. Put the veggies on a grill tray and season with salt and pepper. Cook, turning constantly, until the edges are brown.
5. Cook the chicken about 4 to 5 minutes on each side, until grill marks appear. Transfer to a platter with the veggies and serve.

Nutritional:

Serving Size	3 oz chicken	1 cup vegetables	
Calories	290	Carbohydrates	8g
Fat	16g	Fiber	3g
Protein	28.5g	Sugar	3.5g
Cholesterol	83mg	Sodium	145mg

Lime and Garlic Marinated Pork Chops

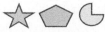

Prep Time: 5 minutes
Cook Time: 10 minutes
Yield: 4 servings

Ingredients:
4 cloves garlic, crushed
½ tsp cumin
4 - 6 oz lean pork chops, boneless
½ tsp chili powder
½ lime, juiced
½ tsp paprika
1 tsp lime zest
1 tsp kosher salt and pepper

Directions:
1. Trim the fat off the pork chops.
2. In a large bowl, season the pork chops with the garlic, chili powder, paprika, cumin, and salt/pepper to taste. Squeeze in the lime juice and some of the zest from the lime. Let it marinade at least 20 minutes or longer.
3. To broil: line a broiler pan with aluminum foil. Place the pork chops on the pan and broil 4 to 5 minutes on each side, or until browned.
4: To grill: grill over medium-high heat 4 to 5 minutes on each side.

Nutritional:

Serving Size	1 pork chop		
Calories	224	Carbohydrates	1.8g
Fat	6g	Fiber	0g
Protein	38g	Sugar	0g
Cholesterol	112mg	Sodium	368mg

Zoodles with Pesto and Tomatoes

Prep Time: 30 minutes
Yield: 4 servings

Ingredients:
For pesto:
1 clove garlic
1 cup fresh packed basil
3 Tbsp extra virgin olive oil
¼ cup fresh grated parmesan cheese
Kosher salt and pepper to taste
For zoodles:
21 oz (3 medium or 4 small) zucchinis
1 cup grape or cherry tomatoes, halved
Kosher salt and black pepper
Directions:
1. Using a food processor, pulse the garlic, basil, parmesan cheese, and salt/pepper to taste, until smooth.
2. While continuing to pulse, slowly add the olive oil. Set the mixture to the side.
3. Spiralize the zucchini. Cut into smaller strands if too long. Place them in a bowl.
4. Toss with the pesto and tomatoes. Add the salt and pepper to taste.
Nutritional:

Serving Size	1 ¼ cups		
Calories	148	Carbohydrates	9g
Fat	12g	Fiber	3g
Protein	4g	Sugar	3g
Cholesterol	4mg	Sodium	102mg

Skillet Steak with Mushrooms and Onions

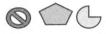

Yield: 4 servings

Ingredients:
½ pound thinly sliced beef round or sirloin steaks
½ large onion, sliced into rings
8 oz sliced mushrooms
½ tsp olive oil
Garlic powder to taste
Non-stick cooking spray
Salt and pepper to taste

Directions:
1. Slice the beef round or sirloin steaks into strips
2. Season with the garlic powder, and salt/pepper to taste
3. Heat a large skillet over high heat. Once hot, spray with the cooking spray and add half of the beef.
4. Cook for one minute, turn steak and cook an additional 30 seconds.
5. Set steak aside in a large dish
6. Spray the skillet again and when it gets hot, add the remaining steak. Cook one minute, turn, and cook an additional 30 seconds. Add to the dish.
7. Return the skillet to the heat, spraying again with the spray. Add the onions and season with salt/pepper. Cook one minute, then turn and cook the onions an additional 30 seconds or until onions are golden brown.
8. Lower the heat to medium and add the olive oil. Put the mushrooms in the skillet. Cook 1 ½ minutes, turning the mushrooms and cooking an additional 1 ½ minutes.
9. Add to the dish with the steak and onions. Stir to combine.
10. Serve over noodles or rice.

Nutritional:

Serving Size	Approx. 4 oz		
Calories	95.4	Carbohydrates	3.5g
Fat	4.1g	Fiber	1g
Protein	12.5g	Sugar	1.1g
Sodium	26.8mg		

Rosemary Broiled Salmon

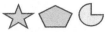

Yield: 4 servings

Ingredients:
24 oz or 4 pieces salmon
2 tsp fresh lemon juice
Olive oil spray
2 cloves garlic, minced
2 tsp fresh rosemary, chopped
Salt and pepper to taste

Directions:
1. Combine the lemon juice, salt/pepper, garlic, and rosemary. Brush the mixture onto the fish.
2. Spray the rack of a broiler pan with the oil spray, arranging the fish on it.
3. Broil fish 4" from the heat until the fish flakes easily with a fork. 4 to 6 minutes per half-inch thickness. Flip halfway through for fish thicker than one inch.

Nutritional:

Serving Size	1 piece		
Calories	245	Carbohydrates	1g
Fat	11g	Fiber	.1g
Protein	34g	Sugar	0g
Sodium	74.5mg	Cholesterol	94mg

Chicken and Avocado Soup

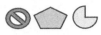

Prep Time: 5 minutes
Cook Time: 20 minutes
Yield: 4 servings

Ingredients:
1 ½ cups scallions, finely chopped
2 tsp olive oil
5 cups reduced-sodium chicken broth
2 cloves garlic, minced
2 small Hass avocados, diced
2 cups chicken breast, shredded
1/3 cup chopped cilantro
1 medium tomato, diced
4 lime wedges
$^1/_8$ tsp cumin
Kosher salt and pepper to taste
Pinch chipotle chile powder

Directions:
1. Using a large pot over medium heat, add the oil, garlic, and one cup of the scallions. Sauté for 2 to 3 minutes until soft. Add the tomatoes and continue for another minute.
2. Add chicken stock, chile powder, cumin, and bring to a boil. Cover and simmer on low for about 15 minutes.
3. In four bowls, add ½ cup chicken, ½ of a small avocado, cilantro, and remaining scallions. Ladle 1 cup chicken broth over the mixture. Serve with lime.

Nutritional:

Serving Size	1 bowl		
Calories	297	Carbohydrates	14.5g
Fat	14g	Fiber	7.5g
Protein	31g	Sugar	2.5g
Sodium	789.5mg	Cholesterol	72.5mg

Roasted Broccoli Parmesan

Prep Time: 5 minutes
Cook Time: 30 minutes
Yield: 4 servings

Ingredients:
1 medium bunch (approx. 20 oz) broccoli with stems
2 Tbsp extra virgin olive oil
6 cloves garlic, peeled and smashed
1 cup homemade or jarred marinara sauce
½ tsp kosher salt
½ cup shredded mozzarella cheese

Directions:
1. Preheat oven to 450°F, grease a 13 x 9 baking dish, and set to the side
2. Trim about one inch of the broccoli stems off the bunch and discard. Slice the stalks in half twice to create four pieces.
3. Place the broccoli, garlic cloves, and drizzle with the olive oil, seasoning both sides of the salt and pepper. Roast cut side down up about 10 minutes. Turn the broccoli and garlic and roast an additional 10 minutes until browned and tender.
4. Top with marinara and mozzarella. Put back into the oven and bake until hot and the cheese is melted, approx. 10 minutes.

Nutritional:

Serving Size	1 piece		
Calories	168	Carbohydrates	13g
Fat	10.5g	Fiber	5g
Protein	9g	Sugar	2g
Sodium	397mg	Cholesterol	11mg

Pass on Dessert

You can scour the web looking for a sweet yet sugar-free treat. Unfortunately, you will be graced with every artificial sweetener under the sun. Some of these claim to be "natural," but when you really look into them, they are manufactured and don't come straight from the source.

I was going to try to give you some kind of dessert to hang your hope on, but the more I looked, the more I realized that it would only be false hope I provided you with. I've made my own changes, a lot of which don't consist of desserts. Sure, you can grab a box of sugar-free pudding and unsweetened almond milk and have at it. A bit of advice if you go that route, you only need about one ¼ cup of almond milk, not the full two you would use with the normal directions. Yes, mistakes were made. Pudding soup definitely has an interesting consistency.

Keeping Your Meal Planning Simple

Sometimes I find myself most stressed about how I'm going to find the time to cook dinner. With a special sugar-free lifestyle, I can't just open a can or whip up something super quick most times. Eating out is also very hard to accommodate, so I do recommend cooking things ahead of time. You can even use your crockpot for cooking meats during the day while you are at work. Then when you get home, you are greeted with tender meat and the smell of success.

Most of the recipes included have "make-ahead" availability to them, especially the breakfast options. Breakfast is often the meal everyone is rushed through, but it is important to get that fuel in first thing. Options like mini quiche or egg muffins provide a powerful protein punch, which helps sustain energy better than a fruity cereal can.

Try New Things

Even if you look at the recipes included and slightly gag, give it a try. You might be surprised that your taste will change some when you aren't constantly dosing it with sugar. I found that the more I stick to the lower carbohydrate and higher protein type menu, the more energy I have during the day. I'm also more satisfied after a meal. I know your next question – yes, the sweet tooth urge will subside after you eat.

You have to keep an open mind when planning your meal approach now. Not every item that will fit best in the sugar-free lifestyle looks appealing, but I promise you are likely to want to try it more than once. Just know that looks can be deceiving!

Fridge, Freezer, and Pantry Staples

There are some foods that you should keep in your refrigerator, freezer, and pantry to be successful limiting your sugar. When you throw out all the old, you can replace it with sugar-free detox friendly alternatives. You will want to make sure you have things on hand to snack on, especially if your cravings get rough.

Refrigerator

Dairy Products
- ☐ Cheddar cheese
- ☐ Butter
- ☐ Cream cheese
- ☐ Cottage cheese
- ☐ Hummus
- ☐ Heavy whipping cream
- ☐ Mozzarella cheese
- ☐ Ricotta cheese
- ☐ Parmesan cheese
- ☐ Sour cream
- ☐ Yogurt, plain, unsweetened

Fresh Vegetables
- ☐ Cauliflower
- ☐ Carrots
- ☐ Cucumbers
- ☐ Limes
- ☐ Lemons
- ☐ Onions
- ☐ Mushrooms
- ☐ Romaine lettuce
- ☐ Shallots
- ☐ Scallions
- ☐ Sweet peppers
- ☐ Spinach
- ☐ Zucchini
- ☐ Tomatoes

Fresh Fruit

- [ ] Blueberries
- [ ] Avocados
- [ ] Cherries
- [ ] Oranges
- [ ] Grapes
- [ ] Nectarine
- [ ] Pears
- [ ] Peaches
- [ ] Plums

Other Staple Fridge Must-Haves

- [ ] Coconut milk
- [ ] Almond milk, unsweetened
- [ ] Deli meat
- [ ] Bacon
- [ ] Garlic
- [ ] Eggs
- [ ] Ground beef
- [ ] Ground turkey
- [ ] Olives
- [ ] Mustard
- [ ] Salsa
- [ ] Pickles
- [ ] Sugar-free ketchup
- [ ] Sugar-free salad dressing

Freezer

- [ ] Frozen berries
  - o Strawberries
  - o Raspberries
  - o Blueberries
  - o Blackberries
- [ ] Frozen leafy greens
  - o Kale

- o Spinach
- o Swiss chard
- □ Frozen vegetables
  - o Broccoli
  - o Carrots
  - o Cauliflower
- □ Turkey, beef, or veggie burgers
- □ Low carbohydrate frozen bread, bagels, waffles, and tortillas
- □ Frozen grilled chicken breasts
- □ Frozen fish fillets

Pantry Essentials

Baking Items
- □ Arrowroot powder
- □ Carob chips
- □ Baking powder
- □ Chocolate, unsweetened
- □ Sugar-free chocolate chips
- □ Xanthan gum
- □ Cocoa powder, unsweetened
- □ Peppermint extract
- □ Vanilla extract
- □ Lemon extract

Beans (canned or dry)
- □ Kidney beans
- □ Cannellini or northern beans
- □ Lentils
- □ Garbanzo beans
- □ Black beans

Breads
- ☐ Whole wheat tortillas
- ☐ Corn tortillas
- ☐ Low carb bread recipes
- ☐ Udi's Gluten-Free Bread

Canned Goods/Jar Items
- ☐ Coconut milk
- ☐ Artichoke hearts
- ☐ Diced tomatoes
- ☐ Crushed tomatoes
- ☐ Low sodium chicken broth
- ☐ Enchilada sauce
- ☐ Olives
- ☐ Sun-dried tomatoes
- ☐ Salsa
- ☐ Tomato sauce
- ☐ Tomato paste
- ☐ Tuna
- ☐ Applesauce, unsweetened
- ☐ Jam, no sugar added

Condiments
- ☐ Sugar-free barbeque sauce
- ☐ Sugar-free ketchup
- ☐ Mustard
- ☐ Dijon mustard

Grains
- ☐ Millet
- ☐ Gluten-free flour
- ☐ Rolled oats
- ☐ Oat bran
- ☐ Popcorn kernels
- ☐ Steel-cut oats

- White whole wheat flour
- Wheat germ
- Whole wheat pastry flour
- Coconut flour
- Almond flour
- Whole wheat flour

Nuts, Seeds, Nut Butters, Seed Butters

- Almonds
- Pumpkin seeds
- Cashews
- Almond butter, unsweetened
- Coconut butter
- Peanut butter, unsweetened
- Hazelnuts
- Pecans
- Walnuts
- Sunbutter
- Peanuts
- Quinoa
- Sesame seeds
- Flaxseed
- Chia seeds
- Sunflower seeds
- Tahini

Oils

- Extra virgin olive oil
- Coconut oil
- Avocado oil
- Ghee
- Nonstick cooking spray
- High heat sunflower oil
- Sesame oil

Spices, Seasonings

- ☐ Cayenne peppers
- ☐ Allspice
- ☐ Celery seed
- ☐ Curry powder
- ☐ Chili powder
- ☐ Cream of tartar
- ☐ Dried oregano
- ☐ Dried basil
- ☐ Dried thyme
- ☐ Italian seasoning
- ☐ Fennel seed
- ☐ Ground cinnamon
- ☐ Garlic powder
- ☐ Ground cumin
- ☐ Ground mustard
- ☐ Ground nutmeg
- ☐ Onion powder
- ☐ Minced onion
- ☐ Pepper
- ☐ Paprika
- ☐ Sea salt
- ☐ Red pepper flakes

It is possible that you will never use half the items on this list, and that is okay. The point of this list is to help you shop and have an idea of the things that fit nicely within the detox program. Seasoning will be one of those important components that can change your meals from drab to fab.

Buy a Little Here – Buy a Little There

When you begin shopping for your new and improved cooking space, keep in mind that you don't have to go out and spend thousands of dollars all at once. Pandemic willing, these items should be available when you go to purchase them.

Start with what you need to make dinner this week and next week. Once you buy some of the versatile items like spices, you don't have to worry about buying them again until you are out. If you mix up your menu each week, you can begin to accumulate quite the collection.

Don't put yourself in a bind starting out. You might end up overwhelming yourself more trying to make sure your pantry and fridge are "just so," instead of a fun learning experience. That's right; I called it fun. You can make your meal planning and grocery shopping for fun.

If you have younger kids, you can get them involved. Plan out a grocery scavenger hunt. The new items may not be something they are familiar with seeing in the house, so it will truly be an epic adventure for them at first.

If you don't have kids, you can make the grocery store your own grown-up scavenger hunt. The same philosophy applies because you aren't used to purchasing these items either!

Learning How to Make It

Once you have been addicted to something, recovery will always be something you have to work at. There are going to be many friends and foes along the way that can either help you or hurt you in your journey. I want to give you a piece of advice, especially when it comes to eating less added sugars – the media is not your friend.

How many times have you seen a commercial and thought about how good the food in the advertisement sounded? This subliminal message is done on purpose. Companies and advertising agencies create ads to prey on those emotions relating to food, such as anxiety, cravings, and addiction.

Anxiety Driven Marketing

Sadly, advertisers know that feelings of anxiety will prompt a situation where people will seek out something to comfort them. One of the most commonly used comforts – food. Not healthy food either, the type full of sugar and void of any real nutritional value.

The Anxiety Disorders Association of America states that two-thirds of those suffering from eating disorders also suffer from an anxiety disorder. When food is used to alleviate anxiety, then it creates a dependency for it, often resulting in poor nutrition.

Cravings and Addiction Through Advertising

Due to the effect of sugar on the brain and the reward receptors, we often crave more and more, never quite satisfied. Marketing ads can play on this part of your brain, showing you images and storylines that pique your interest.

That isn't the only way they play on your emotions. Have you ever been to the supermarket, and they offer you a sample? You know the sample I'm talking about, tiny cup with a small spoon – just enough to draw you in, leaving you wanting another taste. You are baited at that point, purchasing a box, or five, to satisfy what was just awakened.

How about coupons? I love coupons. I can save fifty cents on a candy bar if I buy three just like it! Cha-ching! What did I really save, though? Most of the coupons for food are for the wrong foods. Cereals loaded with added sugar, candy bars, yogurts, etc. You don't see a coupon in the Sunday paper for a dollar off a bunch of kale or seventy-five cents off sugar-free ANYTHING!

HOOK. LINE. SINKER. Just like that – you are hooked.

Even Television Lures You In

How many times have you turned on the television only to see a baking contest or a dessert show? It is these types of shows that promote the idea that sugar is a societal norm. A societal norm is an unwritten rule or behavior that is followed by social groups and culture. It isn't addressed in these shows that sugar, when eaten in excess, can cause various types of diseases up to and including obesity.

We see these commercials and television shows and the celebrities that promote them. We want to be just like them because that is what we are told to do. So when they say they eat donuts for breakfast every morning, then we do the same. Their waist slims down, and ours explodes. What is going on?

You should always approach television as unrealistic. Even reality television is often scripted to some extent. These celebrities are not stuffing their faces full of refined and added sugars, they are likely on the two carrots and kale shake twice a day "diet." Not all celebrities lie about these things, but they get paid to advertise.

If you were offered a $10 million contract to promote using glue sticks as lipstick, you would do it. It doesn't mean that you would actually use the glue sticks anywhere else but in the commercials and promotions, but you would still promote it. Celebrities do this with sugar too.

Recognize and Move Forward

Now you know that these lures are out there, waiting to snatch up some unsuspecting sugar addict (or recovering sugar addict). Recognize them the next time you turn on the television, go to the store, and open up the newspaper. You are stronger than you give yourself credit for.

Think of it as a mindfulness exercise. Acknowledge the bait, and don't judge it. Allow it to move past you, letting you go back to what you were doing before it entered your realm of thought. I won't say that it will be easy to accomplish, but with practice, you can master it.

Change Your Surroundings

I'm not talking about moving out of the country. I'm talking about being able to recognize and move forward, supporting it by removing yourself from specific situations. If you find yourself being tempted by the bakery at the grocery store, you can walk away from it. Go down an aisle with fresh fruits, grab a bag of oranges. Despite being somewhat high in natural sugar, these are better and healthier than a cupcake or a pint of ice cream.

Bittersweet Facts About Sugar

- The typical diet in the United States consists of high sugar sources such as fruit drinks, soft drinks, flavored yogurt, cookies, cereals, candy, cakes, and processed food.
-
- Added sugar is often used to enhance sweetness or to extend a product's shelf life.

- A study that was published in 2014 found that those who have a diet high in added sugar are at a greater risk of dying from heart disease. People who got 17% to 21% of their calories from added sugar had a 38% higher risk of dying from cardiovascular disease when compared to those with only an 8% added sugar calorie intake.

- It has been proven that high-added sugar intake is responsible for inflammation, high blood pressure, weight gain, fatty liver disease, and diabetes. All of these are linked to an increased risk of heart attack and stroke.

- It is possible to consume your entire daily dietary allotment of added sugar by drinking one 12-ounce can of soda.

- The best way to monitor your added sugar intake is to look at the nutrition label for:
  - Corn sweetener
  - Fruit juice concentrates
  - Honey
  - Malt sugar
  - Brown sugar
  - Corn syrup
  - High-fructose corn syrup
  - Invert sugar
  - Molasses
  - Syrup sugar molecules that end in "ose" – dextrose, fructose, glucose, lactose, maltose, sucrose
- A CDC survey ranked the areas where added sugar intake has the highest percentages. They wanted to know where added sugar in our diets comes from.

You might be surprised to know that we drink 42.2% of our added sugar, which was number one on their list.

I'm here to tell you that you do not have to become a statistic. You don't have to "accept" that you are destined to be overweight, have a bad heart, or be prone to depression. While genetics does play a moderate role in your tendency for addictive behavior and all the other factors, you still have the ability to overcome if you choose to.

Did I share with you the time I was ready to "accept my fate?"

It was probably five or six years ago, middle of winter. Keep in mind that I was always a little chunkier than what most consider average, so when I stepped on the ice on the steps, there was only one way to go.

Four hours later, I'm fitted with a temporary cast and an appointment with an orthopedic surgeon. Somehow the way my bones broke was going to need surgical intervention. Did I mention that I broke my femur? That's right twenty-something me broke the strongest bone in the human body. I actually broke right above my ankle too, but that isn't as impressive as the femur.

So imagine, if you will, a plaster cast that runs from the tip of the toe all the way up a slightly bent knee and up to almost my waist. The cast was made to where I could be wheeled, or I could use crutches – I preferred to use the couch.

It wasn't like I was active, to begin with; I obviously had some shortcomings in the exercise field. Now with the leg, and in the dead of winter...let's be real.

I sought the comfort of food, mainly sugar, and those creamy, savory treats. Even as my leg began healing and the cast was eventually removed, I found reasons to keep up my bad habits. "Physical therapy made my leg hurt; I need to rest." "It's Friday; I have to rest for the weekend." "It's Monday; I'm tired from the weekend." Do you see a pattern?

I grew comfortable being sedentary. It brought me great comfort, and I embraced it, as did my waistline. Before I knew it, I was tipping the scale at numbers only seen on television shows (not quite, but that was what it felt like). When I realized what I had done to myself, I thought getting healthy again would be too hard. I wanted to accept my fate and be done with it.

Obviously, I powered through those feelings because I'm writing this book. Part of everything I went through is actually part of what fueled my passion to further change my diet. I wanted to feel good for the first time in my life.

So, I guess what I want you to know is that you don't have to be the product of your genetics. I thought I had to be, but then I remembered that I was me – not just some DNA profile.

Chapter Eight: The Truth, The Whole Truth, and Nothing But The Truth (About...)

I wanted to create a chapter dedicated to breaking down the truth about what added sugar does to the body. There are so many vague discussions, but facing the truth can be ugly – I'll apologize in advance.

We know that added sugar is the fuel behind many different illnesses and diseases. While it may not directly cause a lot of them, it is an underlying factor that contributes. I want you to know the truth that the sugar manufacturers won't put in their advertising campaigns.

Understanding the truth of each of these sugary death traps can help you find a little more motivation – your health. I had to have a rude awakening about what I was doing to myself, and when you see what each of these can do to your body, you'll think twice about eating that tub of icing for supper (you know you've done it, there is no use in lying now).

The Truth About Obesity

The belief for so long has been that people who are overweight eat too much, that is why they are obese. The reality is not quite as simple as some want it to be. Roughly 33% of adults and 25% of children in America fall into this category. Obesity has the ability to impact a person's social health and interpersonal relationships. It can also exasperate and facilitate other health conditions, such as:

- Sleep apnea
- Digestive problems
- Type 2 diabetes
- Stroke
- Osteoarthritis
- Gynecological problems
- Sexual problems
- Cancer
- Heart disease

A person who is obese may exhibit symptoms like snoring, binge eating, fatigue, and a potbelly. Classified as a disease, obesity is diagnosed by calculating a person's body mass index (BMI). A person is obese if they fall into ranges that are not considered healthy.

Three Classes of Obesity

A person's BMI is calculated using their height and weight. It can be calculated using an equation, or you can use a chart to see where you fall on the scale. The formula: weight (lb) / [height (in)]^2 x 703, is used to determine your BMI number. A BMI number between 18.5 and 29.9 is considered healthy. Class 1 obesity is a BMI of 30 to 34.9, class 2 is 35 to 39.9, and class 3 is 40 or higher.

The higher the BMI number, the more at risk you are for developing diseases or other obesity-related problems.

Causes of Obesity

Obesity can be influenced by many factors in your life, such as genetics. You are more likely to develop a weight problem if your parents had one. The genetic factor is the gut microbiome. Lifestyle choices, socioeconomic factors, pregnancy, age, stress, lack of sleep, and previous weight loss attempts play a role as well.

Is There a Cure?

Sadly, there is not a one-size-fits-all solution for obesity. What works for one person may not work for another. In most cases, following a diet and exercise regimen based on your body type can increase the odds of losing weight on your own. Cutting out added sugars, carbohydrates, increasing proteins, etc., have been found to be beneficial. That does not mean that you will be able to get yourself to the healthy BMI range, but it does mean that you can reduce your risk of developing illnesses and diseases in the long run.

The Truth About Type 2 Diabetes

There are two primary types of diabetes – Type 1 and Type 2. Type 1 diabetes is associated with the pancreas not producing insulin for the body to regulate blood sugar. These types are not associated with one another. Type 2 is often found in obese people. It is when your body resists the effects of insulin or doesn't produce enough insulin to maintain levels. There is not a cure for type 2 diabetes, but losing weight and exercising may be enough to manage the problem.

Symptoms Associated with Type 2 Diabetes

The signs and symptoms of type 2 diabetes are often slowly onset. You could have type 2 diabetes for years without knowing it. Often found in routine bloodwork, type 2 diabetes can cause a lot of problems for the body's systems.

The symptoms include:

- Frequent urination
- Unintended weight loss
- Blurred vision
- Frequent infections
- Increased thirst
- Increased hunger
- Fatigue
- Slow-healing sores
- Areas of darkened skin, usually around the armpits or neck

Risk Factors of Developing Type 2 Diabetes

You may be at risk for type 2 diabetes if:

- You are overweight – the main risk factor for type 2 diabetes is being overweight

- Your fat storage is primarily in your abdomen – the risk is greater in men and women who store their fat at their waistline versus those who carry it in their hips or thighs
- You are inactive – the less active you are, the more likely you could develop type 2 diabetes
- There is a family history – you are at a higher risk if your parents or siblings have a history of type 2 diabetes
- You are of a certain race or ethnicity – it is not clear why, but people of African American heritage, Hispanic, American Indian, and Asian Americans are at a higher risk of developing type 2 diabetes
- You are older – the risk of developing type 2 diabetes increases as you get older
- You are a prediabetic – prediabetes occurs when your blood sugar level is higher than normal but not high enough to be considered diabetic
- Pregnant women with gestational diabetes – women who experienced gestational diabetes during pregnancy or birthed a child more than nine pounds are more at risk for type 2 diabetes
- History of polycystic ovarian syndrome (PCOS) – women with PCOS are at a higher risk for type 2 diabetes than women who do not have it
- Areas of darkened skin – if you have areas of darkened skin, usually around the armpits or neck, it can indicate an insulin resistance

Consequences of Type 2 Diabetes

Long-term consequences of type 2 diabetes often progress slowly, but there are some serious health problems associated with the disease. The chances of developing these diseases are higher if you do not manage type 2 diabetes early on.

- Heart and blood vessel diseases
- Kidney damage
- Nerve damage, also known as neuropathy
- Eye damage
- Hearing impairment
- Slow healing
- Sleep apnea
- Skin conditions
- Alzheimer's Disease

To prevent these types of illnesses as a result of type 2 diabetes, it is important to implement a diet without added sugar and exercise. Although some problems are unavoidable, you can work on making lifestyle changes now to better your success of not developing type 2 diabetes, especially if you have a high-risk factor of developing it.

A healthy lifestyle includes eating healthier foods, being active at least 30 minutes three to five times a week, losing weight if you are obese, and avoiding being inactive for too long.

The Truth About High Blood Pressure

High blood pressure is called "the silent killer." High blood pressure, or hypertension, is when your blood pumps with too much force against the walls of your arteries. Luckily, high blood pressure can be managed with the right lifestyle changes.

The truth – high blood pressure has almost no symptoms. Short of having your blood pressure checked, you may not even know that you have it. You could be sitting here reading this while your arteries, heart, and other vital organs are being damaged due to high blood pressure. Dramatic? Not at all. There are so many problems that are associated with high blood pressure that can make it a deadly situation.

High Blood Pressure Can Lead to These Serious Diseases

Your blood pressure affects different organs in different ways, which means that high blood pressure affects these same organs in extremely dangerous ways. Some of the more serious complications that can be caused by high blood pressure are:

- Stroke
- Vision loss
- Memory loss
- Angina (heart pain)
- Kidney damage

- Erectile dysfunction
- Fluid in the lungs
- Peripheral artery disease

Understanding Your Blood Pressure

Your blood pressure reading is interpreted as two numbers. The top number, systolic, which measures the pressure when the heart beats while pumping blood. The bottom number, diastolic, measures the pressure when the heart is at rest. Generally, normal blood pressure is represented by a reading of 120/80 or lower.

Don't be too shocked by high blood pressure, though. Nearly half of the adult population in the United States has it (46%). There are risk factors that may make you more prone to developing it.

Risk factors for developing high blood pressure include:
- Age
- Gender
- Smoking
- Diabetes
- Too much alcohol
- Heredity
- Excess weight or obesity
- High cholesterol
- Sedentary lifestyle
- Unhealthy diet

The American Heart Association recommends that those who are at risk of developing high blood pressure do the following:

- Avoid tobacco, including second-hand smoke
- Exercise regularly
- Maintain a healthy weight
- Use a hot tub safely – extreme temperatures can negatively impact blood pressure
- Eat a healthy diet, preferably low-sodium
- Limit alcohol consumption
- Manage stress

If you find that your blood pressure runs high, but you aren't doing any of the above, you may want to start out with a walk three times a week. Something to keep you from being stationary for a long period of time and walking is also great for weight loss. The use of yoga and meditation are great for managing stress – a huge risk factor for increased blood pressure.

What Do These Have in Common?

I chose to give you a more in-depth look at these because they are all connected. They can also be connected to an excessive amount of added sugar. It is a brutally, life-changing cycle of bodily destruction that leads to despair. Ominous right?

Think about it like this; added sugar contributes to excess weight gain. Excess weight gain leads to obesity. Obesity is a common factor in both high blood pressure and type 2 diabetes. There is a common denominator, which can be eliminated for a healthier lifestyle – added sugar!

I would never have thought that so many illnesses could be linked or traced back to the amount of added sugar we eat. I have the risk factors for developing these, and it is hard to think about where I would be if I hadn't changed my lifestyle. Between genetics and obesity, the best thing I did for myself was decide that a cupcake was not worth a coronary.

I found alternative ways to satisfy my cravings – exercise, reading, writing, and other hobbies. I have the belief that you will too!

The Villain in the Scenario

I'm not trying to ruin your outlook on sugar completely. There are still some sugars that occur naturally that fit into a healthy diet. Those found in fruits, for example, have their place in your diet. Even though the body doesn't differentiate between added sugar and naturally occurring sugars, it is the amount that matters.

A good place to start is the food pyramid. Look to see what your servings of fruits, vegetables, and added sugars should be. Again, each person is different, so learning your tolerance may be a trial and error situation.

The goal is to defeat the added sugar villain and allow you to reign as the superhero in this scenario. (Preferably without high blood pressure, obesity, and type 2 diabetes – not superpowers!)

Be an Overcomer

The fact that you could develop these problems because you eat too much sugar is scary. That's right; I'm saying YOU SHOULD BE SCARED. Nobody wakes up in the morning and says, "I am so glad that I have type 2 diabetes and high blood pressure!" You will need someone to bust your chops when you do the sugar detox, especially if you plan on continuing it.

You have what it takes. I want you to know that. Even if you don't believe in yourself, I know that you can be an overcomer. Before I conclude this book, I want you to take a good look in the mirror. Look at how fierce you can be. Seriously, make the most ferocious face you can. You are a warrior!

Roll with the Punches – There will be a lot!

Part of being successful is not dwelling on the failures but learning from them and refusing to make the same mistake again. You don't stay down when you are dealt a hearty blow because you know that you can change your life by staying the course.

Always take it one day at a time and if you find yourself having a bad day, think of all the good things you have accomplished. Use this time to really look at yourself and see where you are headed. You are changing your health, your mind, your body, and your way of thinking. That's pretty extraordinary.

Conclusion: There is Life After Sugar

You started the sugar detox process over 40 days ago. You have experienced so many things during this time, and you may have even thought that you wouldn't make it to see the morning sun. You prevailed, just like I did.

I started this book thinking that I was going to tell my story, give you some resources, and call it a day. I never imagined that it would grow in the way that it has. I never thought that I would become an advocate for those who want to live their life without sugar.

But here I am, your personal cheerleader – hoping that you can continue going the distance. The facts are startling when you look them up. The number of health risks that are caused by excessive amounts of sugar. Sugar! Who would have thought? It was Mary Poppins who sang that a spoonful of sugar helps the medicine go down! Even childhood storylines talk about sugar being a good thing.

At what point do we draw the line on the amount of sugar we eat, drink, consume daily?

Your Body, Your Choice

As much as I want to tell you that you need to do this for yourself, it is ultimately your choice. You alone are the one that has to decide that your health is worth it and that you want to change the way you approach sugar in your life.

I covered a lot of information throughout this book. You are now informed on what medical problems you might encounter if you continue eating an excessive amount of added sugar. I can't predict the future – you may not end up with any of them! Every person's body is different.

Think About Your Current Health

Start by looking at your current meal plan. I am almost willing to bet that you don't keep track of what you eat. If you don't, you aren't paying attention to the amount of sugar, carbohydrates, etc., that you are pouring into your body. You might be surprised and motivated just by starting there.

If you currently suffer from obesity, high blood pressure, type 2 diabetes, kidney problems, or any of the other diseases/illnesses that I have talked about, what do you have to lose by trying this? It is possible that you might be able to sustain a healthier lifestyle by reducing or eliminating the amount of added sugar you have in your diet.

Do This For Yourself

Have you ever felt like you weren't living your best life? Found yourself depressed and suffering from low self-esteem? I urge you to try the 40-day sugar detox plan I have created. Even if you don't completely eliminate all the sugar from your diet, I can almost guarantee that you will see a change in your life if you eliminate the added sugars.

You owe it to yourself (and your family) to work toward a better existence – one where you are thriving and not riddled by any number of illnesses. Take control of your life and start the sugar detox process. Make your plan for living a life that is not controlled by the covert sugar spies lurking around every corner.

Why You Need to Sugar Detox

If I haven't made the reasons clear, the most important reason to detox from sugar is for yourself. Your health should be a priority. With all the research being done on the subject, it is being discovered that any number of illnesses can be linked to an excessive amount of sugar.

I get it. You love cakes and candies. I love cakes, candies, cupcakes, ice cream, and basically anything that has more added sugar than a bag of sugar (addict, remember?). Luckily there are alternatives, ones that stop you from eating a bag of sugar a day while satisfying your cravings.

I never said it would be easy to work through your addiction, but I am cheering you on. Always know that this book is here to help you get through the toughest parts of the process and help you celebrate the victories, no matter how big or how small they might be!

Don't forget to make ample use of the interactive sheets within this book. Use the meal planner to create a menu and a shopping list to accommodate all your sugar-free cuisine needs. Go through the stages and set your goals. Make reasonable rewards for yourself – and make sure you follow through.

Don't Give Up

I know that there will be times that will seem like you can't move forward. That everything you are doing is nothing but a hopeless journey. Trust in the fact that you have the ability to move forward using your new-found lifestyle.

Think of this as an adventure, one that you can do with the ones you love. Did you know that if a child never tasted ketchup, they wouldn't have developed a desire for it? We start children out early with condiments like ketchup, and they develop that sweet tooth for it.

We learned from our parents, who learned from their parents, so it isn't something that we have developed on our own. We are conditioned from an early age to accept added sugar as a societal norm. At what point can we break that cycle, though?

Believe it or not, we would never know what we were missing if we never had it. So why is it that we can't seem to let go of it after we have it? Our brain sees it as a reward, and we revere sugar as a reward. We equate sugar with something good instead of being bad for our health.

Are you ready to take the challenge with me? Are you ready to begin your 40-day sugar detox program and finally change the way your mind and body cope with things like stress, anxiety, and finally overcome the addiction you never knew you had?

Thank you for taking the time to read this book. I hope that you will take my advice and the knowledge that I am bestowing upon you to work each day to living a sugar-free life. You are special, and you owe it to yourself and your family to at least try my methods for clearing sugar from your life.

Review This Book

If you enjoyed reading this book and got a great value from it, I'd like to ask you to leave a review on Amazon. It would help me a lot in spreading word about this book and I would love to read your thoughts! And yes, I read them all.

Download The Audiobook Free!

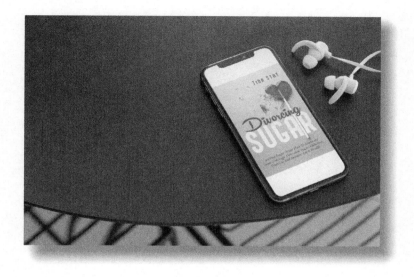

Just to say thanks I would like to give you the
audiobook version 100% free!

To get instant free access go to:
http://www.tinastat.com/audiobook

Printed in Great Britain
by Amazon

25465875R00139